PRAISE FOR

THE PLANT-BASED JOURNEY

"If you're wanting to eat more plants and fewer animals, congratulations! You now have in your hands a trustworthy guide for how to take the journey, step to step, to a more fabulous you. You'll feel better, you'll look better, and you'll enjoy life more. If you accept Lani Muelrath's invitation, your body will thank you for the rest of your life. Highly recommended."

—John Robbins, author *Diet For A New America* and 9 other bestsellers; cofounder and president of The Food Revolution Network

"Let Lani open your eyes with *The Plant-Based Journey*. She deserves your attention."

—John and Mary McDougall, founders of the McDougall Program and authors of *the Starch Solution*

"Lani has created a great 'HOW TO' book for every stage of your plant-based journey. We're also thrilled to see her emphasize how our food choices affect not just our own health but the health of our living planet as well."

—Suzy Amis Cameron and James Cameron

"The journey to evolution and compassion starts with what we eat every day. Read this book and step through the gateway to a new dimension, a whole new world of guilt-free eating and joyous living. As they say, peace begins on your plate."

—Jane Velez-Mitchell, editor or JaneUnChained.com, bestselling author

"Micro changes, restaurant tips, plantify your pantry . . . and so much more. We want the vitality, weight control, and energy that plant based nutrition offers but don't always know how to implement the plan. Lani scores a bull's-eye in *The Plant-Based Journey* by making the process so clear cut and reachable. This is a must-read manual for life."

—Joel Kahn MD, Professor of Medicine, Wayne State University School of Medicine, author of *The Whole Heart Solution*

"Way to go, Lani! You've provided a terrific road map for anyone interested in creating a plant-strong® lifestyle. This easy-to-follow guide will have everyone enjoying the health benefits from following a whole-foods/plant-based diet."

—Rip Esselstyn, author, *The Engine 2 Diet*

"I *love* this book. A fresh, clear, and imminently doable approach to a food-choice upgrade that you can start right now and be in love with by tomorrow. If you're even a bit curious about life on the veg side, Lani Muelrath is the perfect guide for your plant-based journey."

—Victoria Moran, author of *The Good Karma Diet* and director of *Main Street Vegan Academy*

"Lani covers the plant-based journey thoroughly, creatively, and with the exceptional knowledge gained from her years of teaching. When you finish *The Plant-Based Journey*, not only will you be inspired to eat plant based, but you will have the wisdom how to cook the food you enjoy."
—Caldwell B. Esselstyn, Jr., M.D., author of *Prevent and Reverse Heart Disease*

"Lani makes leaning into your healthy transformation so doable. She takes you by the hand and guides you every step of the (wonderful) way with her clear-headed and science-based rationale! Take this journey with her. You will be profoundly changed for the better."
—Kathy Freston, *New York Times* bestselling author of *Veganist* and *The Lean*

"In *The Plant-Based Journey*, Lani Muelrath delivers sound, practical, and essential advice for improving our lives —and the lives of everyone around us. Please get this book and enjoy the adventure of enlivening and awakening your best self."
—Gene Baur, cofounder and president of Farm Sanctuary and bestselling author

"Lani Muelrath's manifesto on healthy living should be a must-read for anyone wanting to get healthy, reach their ideal weight, and stop dieting forever. In her signature accessible style, Lani offers real-life advice for adopting a plant-based diet with ease—complete with stocking your kitchen, dining out tips and tricks, and cooking delicious food the entire family will love. I frequently meet people who want to ditch the meat and take charge of their health, and *The Plant-Based Journey* is the book I will tell them to read."
—Colleen Holland, cofounder of *VegNews Magazine*

"*The Plant-Based Journey* is a flawless, comprehensive, easy-to-follow template for implementation and maintenance of the plant-based lifestyle. Whether for weight loss, concern for human or planetary health, ethics, or simple curiosity, Lani provides the perfect balance of information, validation, and motivational gems. Lani's thoughtful and approachable manner of construction with seamlessly woven strategies is impressive to say the least —of particular significance to educators and organizations at all levels. For the immediate benefit of your own health, and that of our planet, this is the book for you."
—Richard Oppenlander, author *Food Choice and Sustainability* and *Comfortably Unaware*, Director of Inspire Awareness Now, non-profit

"Lani makes research-based information about plant-based living inspiring—not boring! She is a walking testament to health, and I am grateful to have access to her wisdom!"
—Susan Levin, MS, RD, CSSD, director of nutrition education for the Physicians Committee for Responsible Medicine, and board-certified sports dietician

"*The Plant-Based Journey* is the most productive trip you can ever make."
—Howard F. Lyman, author of *Mad Cowboy*

"A fantastically thorough, thoughtful, and inspiring guide for creating the healthy and compassionate life you desire."

—Colleen Patrick-Goudreau, author of *The 30-Day Vegan Challenge*

"As you are thinking of joining the evidence-based journey to buoyant health, genuine compassion, and planetary survival, you have now found in this book your master coach. Experienced, trustworthy, clear, and brilliant, Lani, right at your side, will help you to discover, understand and master this path to freedom, joy, and the fullness of living with ease and delight."

—Hans Diehl, DrHSc, MPH, founder of Complete Health Improvement Program (CHIP) and author of *Health Power*

"As a physician, I have found that there is nothing more vital to a person's health than a whole food, plant-based diet. The problem has been showing my patients how to adopt a plant-based diet—until now. With *The Plant-Based Journey*, Lani Muelrath—living proof that this is the fountain of youth—has taken years of experience showing people how to live a healthy life on a plant-based diet and created the definitive guide. Deeply informative, engaging—and a must-read."

—Garth Davis, MD, author of *Proteinaholic*

"If you find yourself knowing what direction to take but searching for helpful momentum, let Lani and this book be your guide. *The Plant-Based Journey* is a fabulous support tool for finding your confidence as you build self-esteem on the path to a healthy lifestyle."

—Douglas J. Lisle, PhD, coauthor of *The Pleasure Trap*

THE
PLANT-BASED
JOURNEY

PREFACE BY
T. Colin Campbell, PhD, & Howard Jacobson, PhD

THE
PLANT-BASED
JOURNEY

A Step-by-Step Guide
for Transitioning to a Healthy Lifestyle
and Achieving Your Ideal Weight

LANI
MUELRATH

BENBELLA

BenBella Books, Inc.
DALLAS, TX

BenBella

BenBella Books, Inc.
10300 N. Central Expressway
Suite #530
Dallas, TX 75231
www.benbellabooks.com
Send feedback to feedback@benbellabooks.com

Printed in the United States of America
10 9 8 7 6 5 4 3 2 1

LCCN: 2015011010
978-1-941631-36-2 (paperback)
978-1-942952-09-1 (electronic)

Editing by Heather Butterfield
Copyediting by Karen Levy
Proofreading by Kimberly Broderick
    and Michael Fedison
Photo on page 241 by LUMI Photography
Indexing by JigSaw Indexing Services
Text design and composition by Kit Sweeney

Front cover design by Bradford Foltz
Jacket design by Sarah Dombrowsky
Printed by Lake Book Manufacturing
Recipes on pages 196, 205, and 209 by
    Miyoko Schinner
Recipe on page 210 by Colleen Holland
Recipe on page 210-211 by Chef AJ

Distributed by Perseus Distribution
www.perseusdistribution.com

To place orders through Perseus Distribution:
Tel: (800) 343-4499
Fax: (800) 351-5073
E-mail: orderentry@perseusbooks.com

Significant discounts for bulk sales are available. Please contact Glenn Yeffeth at glenn@benbellabooks.com or (214) 750-3628.

To everyone on, beginning, or thinking about the journey—

I wrote this book for you.

CONTENTS

PREFACE

As my son Tom and I signed the contract, I knew *The China Study* wasn't going to sell a lot of copies. Turned down by a dozen publishers who knew the market cold, the manuscript was accused of being "too full of science" for ordinary readers. Its message was too far out of the mainstream to be convincing. And, the kiss of death, it was a food book without recipes.

So when a small Texas publishing house, BenBella Books, took on the orphan manuscript in 2004, my expectations were modest. At best, I hoped, it might find its way into the hands of a few serious policy makers and science bigwigs, and thereby influence public discussion in a roundabout way. After all, the weight of evidence favoring a whole food, plant-based diet was overwhelming. The challenge, I thought, was just getting people to see the truth.

I was neither delusional nor imaginative enough to have foreseen what happened next. From a slow start, *The China Study* has now sold over one million copies worldwide. My work and that of the colleagues we profiled in the book have been brought to even wider audiences thanks to films like *Forks Over Knives*.

Now I had another puzzle on my hands. If *The China Study* was so convincing, and it was reaching an audience in the millions, then why was the world so slow to change?

We know that:

- consumption of animal products is clearly linked to unhealthy weight, disease, disability, and untimely death;

- industrial-scale animal agriculture is the single biggest contributor to the most imminent threats to our environment, including climate destabilization, drawdown of our aquifers, and the rise of antibiotic-resistant "superbugs"; and

- our meat-heavy Western diet promotes cruelty to other life forms and to economically and politically disadvantaged humans.

So why on earth wasn't the message, now widely heard, changing our food system more quickly and systemically?

Nine years after *The China Study*, I published *Whole: Rethinking the Science of Nutrition* (also with BenBella, a loyal partner for all these years) to explain what I thought was holding us back. I identified two main obstacles: all the moneyed interests exerting "subtle power" on the system, and a mind-set that elevated unrelated facts at the expense of large, observable patterns.

My background is in biochemical and epidemiological exploration, with an unavoidable minor in public policy due to my decades of trying to convince political functionaries to create policy based on science, not corporate largesse or threat. *Whole* explored both of those domains in its answer and prescription. Yet there was a companion book to be written—and I wasn't the one to write it—about how people can move from understanding to action.

While I'm no expert on behavior change, I know firsthand (and have heard personal stories from literally thousands of people) that there's a big difference between *knowing* about the benefits of a plant-based lifestyle and actually *living* it. So when my *Whole* contributing author and cowriter of this preface, Howard Jacobson, told me that Lani Muelrath was working on the book you now hold in your hands, I knew it was the companion volume to *Whole* that needed to be written.

Lani has been on the plant-based journey far longer than we have (decades, in fact, before I coined the phrase "whole food, plant-based" to describe more accurately than "vegan" the dietary pattern shown to promote individual and global well-being). As she humbly writes, she's made all the mistakes so you don't have to.

It's one thing to have a guide who's already mastered the path you're about to walk; it's another thing entirely when that guide has devoted herself to understanding how and when and why people succeed and how and when and why they stumble. Lani's own transition to a whole food, plant-based lifestyle and subsequent health, energy, and fitness are admirable and instructive. But it's her experience coaching thousands from initial awakening to unconscious competence that makes her a powerful partner on your own plant-based journey.

As researchers, we have long love affairs with valid data and validated theories. We're happy to report that this book contains both. Not only has Lani scoured the medical and nutritional literature to present her case for a plant-based diet, but she has also devoured the literature on habit formation and behavior change, exercise physiology and brain function, and psychological processes of decision making.

The most useful data, however, comes from Lani's own research. She surveyed over 1,200 people at various stages of the plant-based journey to discover what they found helpful, what strategies did and didn't work, and what advice they'd give to someone just about to take the first step.

This book represents the culmination of their combined experience with Lani's wisdom, compassion, humor, and "just the facts" outlook. If you are just starting out, or finding yourself struggling to eat in accord with your knowledge and your values, or looking to take your plant-based game to the next level, then *The Plant-Based Journey* is your new best friend.

We wish you abundance, harmony, and joy on your plant-based journey.

—T. Colin Campbell, PhD, and Howard Jacobsen, PhD

FOREWORD

So much has happened in the past few decades to fuel the fire of the plant-based movement, and it has been very exciting to see things unfold. Since the founding of the Physicians Committee back in 1985, we have been conducting clinical research studies to test the effects of eating a low-fat vegan diet on health. We have consistently found that this way of eating brings benefits in a wide range of health areas. One of our biggest studies, funded by the National Institutes of Health, was conducted with people who had type 2 diabetes, and the results were impressive. A plant-based diet was found not only to be even more effective than a more conventional "diabetes diet," but it also was more powerful than oral diabetes medications. Many of our study participants were able to completely get off of their medications or significantly reduce the amount of their daily dose(s). In our numerous studies on diabetes since then, the outcome has been the same. A low-fat vegan diet bas been shown to be therapeutic for myriad conditions in numerous other research studies conducted through our organization and many others. For everything from heart disease to migraines, depression to arthritis, plants have proven to be powerful mechanisms for healing the body and promoting health.

When people participate in our research studies, it is typical for that to be their first encounter with eating a plant-based diet. Accordingly, they need some guidance on how to get started and integrate this new diet into their current lifestyle. Thankfully, we have a wonderful group of staff members on our clinical research team who are full of knowledge and have years of experience to share. And once our participants get the first few weeks under their belts (which by that point may likely be a little looser than when they started), they'll have fallen into an eating pattern that will feel almost second nature. Although it may be hard to believe right now, in time, a plant-based diet will feel like home—natural, easy, and right—but getting there is a journey.

Like our research participants, you, too, may need some guidance as you're getting started. Lucky for you, you have Lani to help you. She escorts you through the transition step by step, offering valuable support and advice along the way. For everything from restocking your kitchen to eating on the road, Lani helps you to steer through the obstacles like a pro. So, are you ready to take the wheel? With a book like this in your hands, the answer is yes!

Buckle up and enjoy the ride. The plant-based journey takes you to the very best of places.

—Neal Barnard, MD

INTRODUCTION

In Gary Larsen's classic *There's a Hair in My Dirt*, the story's heroine, Harriet, has a series of encounters with wildlife while on a day's walk in the woods: a tortoise on the trail, a fledgling bird fallen from its nest. In her heartfelt compassion for the natural world, Harriet innocently tries to help, yet with disastrous results. She tosses the tortoise into a pond, mistaking its needs for that of a water-going turtle, thus sending it to its doom. She scales a tree to place the chick back into its nest, not understanding that the survival of just one offspring is critical to the entire species' survival. Harriet is brimming with caring and compassion for the natural world. Yet while earnest about making a positive difference, she lacks the practical knowledge about how to be most helpful. This results in her repeatedly thwarting the desired outcomes of her endeavors.

In similar fashion, you may be bubbling over with enthusiasm for the plant-based lifestyle. Perhaps you've been freshly inspired—or have renewed passion about—your health, your weight, the environment, and the significant difference a plant-based lifestyle can make for it all. This inspiration has brought you to this juncture and underpins your quest. Just like Harriet, you care! And caring is the place from where any change necessarily springs forth.

Where you may need a boost—just like Harriet—is in the practical, personal connection portion of the program. This is exactly what you'll find in this book. The highly successful model for your quest—*The Plant-Based Journey*—is drawn from over four decades of both personal practice and experience coaching thousands on their successful transitions to the healthy plant-based lifestyle. This journey invites you to center what you eat on predominantly whole plant foods: vegetables, whole grains, beans and legumes, fruits, nuts, and seeds. There are straightforward, sound, proven ways to set yourself up for successful transition. They are simple to learn and easy to implement, and they are assembled for you here. You'll discover how to keep it uncomplicated, inexpensive, doable, and delectable. You'll find out how to leverage simple systems that support your new ideal. We'll also dismantle and clear away obstacles that may be getting in your way—for the conventions of eating extend to beyond just what you're used to putting on your plate.

THE JOURNEY'S PATH

When people come to me for help in changing to a plant-based diet, many times they ask questions about nutrition and meal ideas. Yet even more often they have become tangled in the transition. They need practical guidance to help them not only set up their kitchen but also unravel their previous practices of eating—and thinking. They are often at the juncture between knowing enough about the shortfalls, compromises, and serious hazards of continuing to eat in the fashion they have been, sincerely desiring something better for themselves—yet floundering when it comes to making the shift. Without practical knowledge of some basics, along with being properly equipped with the tools needed for real, lasting change, they, like Harriet, inadvertently impair their success. For food—beyond providing us with good nutrition—is also about habits, family, friends, workplace, travel, social situations, traditions, and comfort. How do you successfully navigate all of that?

This is where the steps as spelled out for you in *The Plant-Based Journey* come in. Though each of us brings a uniqueness to the journey of changing to eating a plant-based diet, there are universal stages along the way, which are explained below. Think of them as levels of proficiency through which your expedition will progress. There are no set intervals, no rules of pace on the journey through each of these stages. Progression through them is an individual affair.

Section One: Awakening

This is the first stage you will go through in transitioning to a plant-based diet. Everyone starts this journey as the result of an inspiration. Some event, person, or circumstance has alerted you to a new way of looking at what you eat. You have, literally, become awakened to a new possibility—the plant-based lifestyle. Awakening is what gives your journey its first legs and is the single most important element of transition. In section one, we'll establish a quick reconnect with your reasons for embarking on this journey—your "why."

Section Two: Scout

In section two, we'll focus on plant-based eating basics. This is the investigative stage, where those initial questions and curiosities are addressed. What does a plant-based lifestyle look like in your kitchen, in your shopping cart, and on your plate? How do you morph your current shopping, cooking, and eating styles to align with your new ideal, and avoid common pitfalls? What food preparation tools will help make the whole thing easier? As Scout, you are gathering information. It's a reconnaissance mission.

Section Three: Rookie

Soon emerging, and often overlapping with the Scout stage—because you will no doubt be inspired to start eating more whole plant foods while still in the investigative process—is the Rookie stage. Here, you apply the knowledge from Scout reconnaissance to specific action. It's time to eat! You'll strategically increase the presence of plant foods on your plate and create simple systems for successful implementation, crowding out animal products and highly processed foods. Quite quickly, what used to feel awkward you now find yourself accomplishing with ease. Soon you are eating plenty of plant-based foods each day to make and keep you healthy, happy, satisfied, and trim.

Section Four: Rock Star

When 90 percent of your calories come from a variety of whole, plant-based foods, you've clearly achieved Rock Star status. You continue to sharpen the tools of expertise with greater confidence and ease and are inspired to evolve your plant-based practices onto a bigger stage. That means preparedness for travel, vacations, a busy work schedule, and restaurant dining—not to mention those family and social situations that seem to present themselves at every turn. Increasingly, you'll build the skills for making the practical connection between what you *know* about a plant-based lifestyle and what you *do*.

Section Five: Champion

As Champion, at ease with the basics, you've also assembled and are consistently practicing strategies for flourishing in a healthy, happy, plant-based lifestyle. Now that you are eating predominantly whole plant foods, you have new know-how for some of the more complex challenges of the journey. At this level, you'll leapfrog your enjoyment and expertise for successful lifestyle longevity.

Section Six: The Key Supporting Players: Exercise and Mastering Strength of Mind

In this section you'll find out how physical activity and mobilizing your mind for change add enormous oomph to your journey. Together, they poise you for positive transformation, enhancing brain function and setting you up for making better choices—while dismantling hidden obstacles and increasing ease, satisfaction with, and sustainability of your plant-based lifestyle.

. . .

Throughout these six sections, we'll restore your birthright—the pure joy of eating. Food is meant to be relished with gusto, free of overstructured artifice, bodily discomfort, disease, cognitive dissonance, or a looming threat of weight gain. When you take back your fork, you reclaim your freedom. Your body and beltline will thank you forever.

You may be completely new to this journey or in the middle of any of the above stages. Excellent! Simply step in and move forward from wherever you are. Dip back as needed into previous stages to refresh your know-how. This has the effect of elevating your journey and averting black-and-white thinking—perhaps the number-one downfall of lifestyle change. At every step of the journey—from Awakening to Champion—keep mindful of the fact that the closest thing to perfect is continued overall improvement. What a relief! With this understanding, your journey—already under way with the first signs of Awakening—will be one of brilliant, sustainable success.

MORE LIGHT FOR YOUR JOURNEY'S PATH

While researching this book, I gathered over 1,200 responses to surveys about personal experiences on the plant-based journey. In these surveys, I asked specific questions about what my clients and readers found helped them successfully advance along the plant-based path. I asked them what worked for them, the suggestions they might have for those just setting out, and what they wish they had known *before* they got started. Providing insights and reflections from the front lines of change, these surveys—along with my decades of coaching experience—are referenced, reported, quoted, and otherwise woven into the fabric of this book.

In your hands is the handbook and companion for taking your plate from plant-spare to plant-prolific, and for opening the door to true eating freedom. Excited to get going? Your plant-based journey is now under way.

Devotion and keeping it simple will merrily ferry you through the early stages. With heart, enthusiasm, and a little bit of planning, it will soon become second nature, deeply satisfying—and more fun, rewarding, and liberating than you ever imagined.

AWAKENING

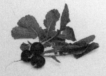

The Adventure Begins

CHAPTER 1
Making the Plant-Based Connection

Your imagination has been captured, your heart won. Whether you want to lose weight, increase day-to-day vigor, lower your cholesterol, reverse or prevent disease, enhance athletic performance, exert less impact on the environment, or simply live in a more compassionate world, the plant-based lifestyle sounds like just what you are looking for. You've awakened to new possibilities. You're primed and ready! In this chapter you will explore the first stage of your plant-based journey—identifying your "why"—underscoring your motivations for eating plant-based.

My guess is that your journey began before you even opened this book. Something you read, someone you talked with, or something you heard has ignited in you the inspiration to recast your lifestyle in a fundamental way: by what you put on your plate. Your reasons for embarking on this journey may be multiple, or you may have one overriding incentive for embracing the plant-based lifestyle. Yet don't be surprised if before long you become aware of a growing list of compelling reasons that support your choice. Cultivate your connection to each of them. Having multiple motivations further energizes your quest.

WHY PLANT-BASED?

Research tells us that the most common reasons people move to eating meat-reduced or meat-free are to improve their health and/or the lot of animals, followed by a concern for the environment.[1] Living a plant-based lifestyle has a positive and powerful impact on all three areas. The truth is that if you can get control of your food, you can get control of more than you ever imagined.

To help you flesh out your purpose in going plant-based, what follows is a snapshot of the common reasons that people make this far-reaching lifestyle change. Rather than providing an exhaustive discourse on reasons for becoming plant-based, the intention of this chapter is to put important information into your hands so that you can make your own informed decisions about the journey, and to underscore the importance of being connected with your "why" for getting started.

We'll start by hitting closest to home—your weight, health, and how you feel in your body.

Weight Loss and the Dietary Holy Grail: You Can Be Full without Being Fat

My own weight challenges spurred me on a decades-long quest to find a way of eating that would allow me to, bottom line, be well fed without being fat. This search finally landed me happily on the whole food, plant-based doorstep. Eating this way has allowed me to easily maintain—while eating to my heart's content—a weight 50 pounds lighter than the one at which I found myself almost twenty years ago. More details in chapter 2.

You'll be relieved to know that there is no reason to shrug off your weight problem—if indeed you have one—as, "it's in my genes." Though it may be, the research tells us that behavior trumps genetics. What you eat has more bearing on your fat or lean condition than do your genes. Predisposition is not destiny. Bestowing vitality and glowing health, a plant-based diet will restore—or help you find for the first time ever—your ideal weight, without you having to chronically go hungry, fanatically exercise, or micromanage every bite. As much as you can certainly be as healthy as possible "at any size," there is a distinct correlation between obesity and advancing disease—to say nothing of the well-being, slender physique, and joy of living that can be yours each day when you make the switch to whole plant foods.

> **TALKING MEAT WITH BILL GATES AND MICHAEL POLLAN**
>
> GATES: Why should people consider replacing meat in their diets?
> POLLAN: Three principal motivators: health, because we know high consumption of red meat correlates with higher chances of certain cancers; the environment, because we know that conventional meat production is one of the biggest drivers of climate change, as well as water and pollution [*sic*]; and ethics, since the animal factories that produce most of our meat and milk are brutal places where animals suffer needlessly.[2]

Troublesome Twosome: Slashing Animal Products and Processed Foods Is Proven to Improve Your Health

Two mealtime monoliths have put our well-being in a precarious position: animal products and highly processed, refined foods. Together, these comprise roughly 90 percent of the calories we, as a nation, consume.[3,4] Both have proven direct links to obesity and disease. A closer look at some of the problems related to eating them will edify your journey.

Americans obtain over 60 percent of their calories in the form of highly processed foods made with refined sugar, oil, and white flour. These show up in pastries, candies, and fast foods, which have hijacked our taste buds with a false "fed" promise—they encourage us to take in far more calories than do whole plant foods to get to our fullness point. In other words, fiber-deficient edibles—as all animal products also are—present problems for hunger satisfaction. Along with other essential nutrients, refined food products have had the fiber ripped out of them. Both are waiting for the fiber absolution that never comes—and animal products never had fiber in the first place. It's not as if nutrients such as fiber are optional for your well-being—they are essential for cellular normalcy and disease protection. When you fraction foods and alter their composition, you change what your body does with them. When the foodstuffs get robbed, so does your health. This also has enormous implications for weight control—more on that in chapter 4 (page 42). Remember, just because it's edible doesn't mean it's food.

The leading causes of degeneration, debilitation, and death in the modern world—heart disease,[5,6] strokes, complications from obesity such as type 2 diabetes, and certain forms of cancer[7]—are largely nutritionally controllable and thus not entirely unavoidable.[8] This means that often you can eat your way out of them through the adoption of a whole plant foods diet.[9,10,11] This has been demonstrated by multiple programs, perhaps the best known being Dr. Ornish's Program for Reversing Heart Disease. Scientifically proven to reverse heart disease, the Ornish program, which includes adoption of a plant-based diet, is currently offered in hospitals and qualifies for coverage by Medicare.[12]   Kaiser Permanente—as an HMO having a decided interest in keeping people healthy—recently issued a directive "to help physicians understand the potential benefits of a plant-based diet, to the end of working together to create a societal shift toward plant-based nutrition."[13] A report by the Union of Concerned Scientists says we could save 100,000 lives and $17 billion annually in health care costs from heart disease if Americans *simply ate more fruits and vegetables.* These are astonishing numbers—and it doesn't stop there (italics my own for emphasis): "If Americans ate just *one more serving* of fruits or vegetables per day, this would save more than 30,000 lives and $5 billion in medical costs each year," and "if Americans were to follow current U.S. Department of Agriculture (USDA) recommendations for daily consumption of fruits and vegetables, those numbers would go up to more than 127,000 lives and $17 billion saved." The report goes on to challenge Congress to slash farm policies that subsidize and thus proliferate Big Ag's massive production of junk and fast food, undeniably contributors to the problem.[14]

Eating More Whole Grains Is Linked with Lower Mortality Risk

Increasing evidence links consumption of whole grains with decreased risk of mortality. Evaluating statistics from more than 100,000 women and men over a period of about twenty-five years, researchers compared the participants' whole grain intake with mortality data. They found that for every serving of whole grains (28g/day), overall death risk dropped by 5 percent, and by 9 percent for cardiovascular disease–related death. The study concludes, "These findings further support current dietary guidelines that recommend increasing whole grain consumption to facilitate primary and secondary prevention of chronic disease, and also provide promising evidence that suggests a diet enriched with whole grains may confer benefits toward extended life expectancy."[15] It's really quite simple. Eat abundantly of whole plant foods and you build a proven protective barrier between you and a landslide of poor health.

Can You Get Too Much?
Animal Protein Intake and Cancer

Too *much* protein? And here you thought we were going to address the plant-based FAQ "where do you get your protein?" In truth, the answer to that question demands a reframing of the entire issue surrounding protein.

There is a distinctly prejudiced attitude that lurks behind the "where do you get your protein?" question. The presumption is that protein is the ultimate macronutrient that we must unquestionably pursue and ingest—and the more of it, the better. This ubiquitous perspective prevails in advertising and oral tradition. "High in protein!" featured on a product label is perceived by the public as an unquestioned positive. Certainly protein plays a crucial role in the structure and functions of the body, having a hand in everything from making muscle to bolstering immunity. No one is arguing that. Yet when it comes to protein, the recommendation for high levels of it in our diet is long outdated and needs to be reevaluated, and our requirements for it based on science rather than special interests.

Actually, most people consume twice the amount of protein needed. Even the Academy of Nutrition and Dietetics (AND) proclaims that "most Americans eat more protein than they need."[16] The recommended dietary allowance (RDA) for protein for both men and women is 0.36 grams per pound of body weight—a little bit more for pregnant or nursing women, easily met with their typical increased calorie consumption. These amounts are in alignment with those recommended by the World Health Organization and AND, and are easily satisfied or surpassed by eating enough calories from a variety of whole plant foods.[17]

A diet of excessive animal protein is correlated with increased risk for multiple health problems and chronic disease.[18] The high-protein habit also hijacks a portion of our plates that should be devoted to plant-produced nutrition while littering our plates with edible land mines. In the heavily referenced, definitive *The Mystique of Protein and Its Implications*,[19] T. Colin Campbell[20] underscores the health risks undeniably linked to our love affair with eating animal protein, which makes it surprisingly easy to surpass our dietary protein requirements for optimal health. Consumption of concentrated protein as found in animal protein increases the body's production of IGF-1—insulin-like growth factor.[21] One of the body's important growth promoters during fetal and childhood development,

IGF-1 normally tapers off after puberty, when our need for growth spurts naturally declines. An elevation in IGF-1 levels later in life promotes the aging process.[22] High levels of IGF-1 have been shown to foster the growth, proliferation, and spread of cancer cells, making IGF-1 a hot topic in oncology.[23,24,25] In contrast, *reduced* IGF-1 in adulthood is associated with diminished oxidative stress, decreased inflammation, enhanced insulin sensitivity, and longer life span.[26,27,28]

The preeminence of animal protein was originally based on the finding that, gram for gram, it promoted more weight gain than did plant-based protein. However, "growing bodies of people faster also means growing cancer faster, both of which are promoted by hormone growth factors."[29] When cancer has been initiated, a high-protein diet that exceeds the amount needed by the body has been shown to promote cancer growth. Casein—the primary protein in milk—has been called "the most 'relevant' chemical carcinogen ever identified."[30] Interestingly, this problem with excess protein pertains only to animal protein, as research has linked diets high in animal protein to the proliferation of cancer—while high amounts of plant protein have not.

In contrast, low-protein diets have been shown to *inhibit* the growth of cancer, without risk to any other aspect of health. *The China Study* concluded, "People who ate the most animal-based foods got the most chronic disease. Even relatively small intakes of animal-based food were associated with adverse effects," while those who ate the most plant-based foods were the healthiest and tended to avoid chronic disease.[31] Distinct correlations also exist between countries with animal protein–rich diets and diseases of lifestyle, such as cardiovascular diseases, and complications from obesity such as diabetes.[32]

Clear correlations have been found between populations that consume low percentages of animal products and proteins and *reduced* incidences of disease.[33] Upon a review of the literature, sixteen scientists from ten countries concluded that diets that are protective against cancer are primarily made up of foods of plant origin.[34] Reducing intake of saturated fats and trans fats—the former found in animal products and both of which are found in refined food products—has been found to reduce the risk of Alzheimer's disease and dementia.[35] No studies documenting an *increase* in lifestyle diseases from eating a whole food, plant-based diet exist.

From Single Nutrients to Whole Foods for Health

The entire isolated nutrients lens through which we've become accustomed to viewing our diet has created a misinformed mind-set about nutrition. "Carbs," "fats," and "protein"—terms that have become the darlings of the processed foods and diet industries—do not accurately inform you about what's in your food. It constructs a can't-see-the-forest-for-the-trees problem, where single nutrients are the individual trees while the entire forest—"wholistic" nutrition—is undervalued and overlooked. This is a convenience for the food supplement industry, which has quite profitably figured out how to leverage our single nutrient obsession with its push of powders and pills. Whole foods can be refined and highly processed to isolate nutrients from their original form of delivery, put in a package, and sold to you at a greatly inflated price in the form of, for example, protein supplements and fatty acid capsules. The cost is even greater when you consider that, in reality, this plant plundering—reducing complex plant foods to emphasize one nutrient—diminishes the nutritional richness of the whole, real thing.

We don't eat nutrients; we eat food. Overanalyzing and dissecting foods in an effort to compartmentalize them by nutrient content sells them short on what they deliver as whole entities—providing the perfect synergy of what you need for optimal nutrition.[36] For example, legumes are more concentrated in amino acids—the building blocks of protein—than many other plant foods. But to call them a protein is an oversimplified misnomer. They are also rich in starch, fiber, vitamins, and minerals. Legumes are not designated to play just one position; their strength—as with other whole plant foods—lies in their ability to play all over the plate, giving them the full court advantage with the superior qualities they quite literally bring to the table.

See Red Meat—and Say No: The Red Meat and Chronic Disease Connection

In 2012, the *Journal of the American Medical Association* issued precautions about including meat on your menu, stating that "consumption of unprocessed and processed red meats is associated with chronic diseases" and "increased risk of total [disease], cardiovascular disease, and cancer mortality."[37] The Harvard School of Public Health publicized these findings that same year, affirming that red meat, especially processed meat, contains ingredients that have been linked to increased risk of chronic diseases, such as cardiovascular disease and cancer.[38]

Chicken and Eggs Increase Disease Risk

Although marketing has driven a "poultry is healthier fare" campaign, chicken has not lived up to the promise. Even in the leanest cuts of chicken, almost 25 percent of the calories are from fat—a hair shy of the 28 percent fat in lean beef—and with just about the same amount of cholesterol.[39] Compare that to beans, rice, and vegetables, which contain an average of 10 to 15 percent calories from fat—*sans* cholesterol.

The public health picture with chicken only gets worse. When it comes to bacteria, chicken is a hot mess. That intestinal "bug" that went around the office last year? Possibly caused by salmonella or campylobacter, fun-sounding bacteria that have been detected on approximately one-third of the chicken products in our supermarkets. Present in the chicken feces, the bacteria is easily splattered onto the skin and muscle tissue during "processing," a polite term for slaughter and evisceration.[40] Sure, you can kill these bacteria with cooking, but you might want to prepare dinner in a hazmat suit.[41]

Cooking chicken presents a problem of its own. Heavily cooked chicken apparently can form cancer-causing chemicals. And these aren't chemical additives—they actually form from the flesh itself sizzling on your seemingly innocent backyard grill.[42] Yikes. And how do you think bird flu epidemics make their way into our population? Domestic bird farms provide perfect breeding grounds for influenza viruses that hitch a ride on migratory birds.

Egg consumption increases the risk of cardiovascular diseases in a dose-response manner—the more you eat, the worse it gets. Researchers discovered that those who consumed the most eggs had a 19 percent increased risk for developing cardiovascular disease and a 68 percent increased risk for diabetes, compared with those who ate the fewest. For those already with diabetes, the risk for developing heart disease from eating the most eggs jumped by 83 percent.[43] Eating eggs is also linked to developing prostate cancer. By consuming 2.5 eggs per week, men increased their risk for a deadly form of prostate cancer by 81 percent, compared with men who consumed less than half an egg per week. Incidentally, the same study revealed a link between red and processed meat and the advancement of prostate cancer.[44]

Peril in the Milk Pail:
The Problems with Dairy Products

Should you just switch out the beef and the chicken for that seemingly innocent "perfect food," milk? Cow's milk can grow a newborn calf to double its weight in about fifty days—in contrast to humans who double birth weight in 180 days.[45] Have we a mismatch?

Dairy products come with their own bucketful of woes—in addition to the issues surrounding casein. Dairy devotees may find that along with the cheese and yogurt come asthma, diarrhea, anemia, arthritis, migraine headaches, allergies, constipation, gas, bloating, eczema, runny nose, acne, and fatigue, along with an elevated risk for a variety of serious illnesses, including type 1 diabetes.[46] On top of all of this, the National Cancer Institute has said, "Milk-drinking is one of the most consistent dietary predictors of prostate cancer in the scientific literature today."[47]

If you step outside the milk carton propaganda, you might find the very idea that the milk of another species is optimal and "needed by every body"—let alone necessary for human health—curious. We know that just the presence of large amounts of calcium in dairy foods consumed doesn't guarantee stronger bones.[48] High intake of cow's milk has even been associated with increased risk for bone fractures and death.[49] A look at the epidemiology around the world reveals that the very countries that consume the most dairy, calcium, and animal protein have the highest rates of osteoporotic bone fracture.[50] And the inverse is so—in countries where they're not obsessed with the milk moustache, we find reduced risk of developing bone disease.[51]

Once you find out some of the contaminants in dairy milk—such as, among other goodies, rocket fuel—you start to rethink it.[52,53,54,55] Simple food web science explains it. Chemicals and pesticides work their way into our waterways, where they are taken up through the roots of plants, which are then eaten by livestock. These substances are sequestered in the animals' fat stores—right along with additional amounts that are applied to crops destined for the dairy cow feedlot. As a dairy cow prepares to make milk, her body mobilizes her fat stores to produce milk for her offspring. This results in the release of chemicals that have been bioaccumulating in the milk—now in a far more concentrated form—which then become exponentially concentrated in the bodies of humans who consume dairy products. What we end up with is a hand-me-down payload of contaminants. This carries lifelong consequences for the humans at the receiving end of dairy products in the form of immune suppressors, carcinogens, and neurotoxins.

Infectious agents taint the milk as well. Somatic cells—white cells and tissue debris, otherwise known as pus—proliferate in the milk supply.[56] This is a "drink your milk!" deal breaker for a lot of people. The fact that white blood cells are showing up in cow's milk is an indication that there's a health problem for the cow. And with the use of antibiotics to control disease in dairy cows, antibiotic residue in milk leads to decreased effectiveness of antibiotics in humans.[57]

BEYOND YOUR BELTLINE: MORE REASONS TO GO PLANT-BASED

The food you eat is arguably the biggest health, medical, environmental, conscience, and sociopolitical decision you make every day. With so much crossover among human health, issues of the environment, and well-founded concerns with livestock raising and "harvesting"—a term loosely used in the meat, poultry, fish, and dairy industries to euphemize the grim reality of the process from feedlot to food purveyor—it can be hard to separate them into different categories of reasons to plant-base your plate.

Proven over and over again to trump heredity and environmental carcinogens[58] while handing back your good health, the plant-based lifestyle also represents the biggest move you can make to reduce the multiple, complex problems directly related to the factory farming of animals.[59] The avalanche of animal products and highly processed edible food-like substances devoured annually not only places our health in peril—it also delivers a deluge of environmental and ethical disasters. Plant-based living is a prescriptive for improvement on all fronts.

Wake Up and Smell the CAFOs: They're Bad News for People and Animals

CAFOs—concentrated animal feeding operations—have been called the biggest offenders when it comes to environmental degradation.[60] Methane emissions from livestock and feedlot runoff pollute our air and waterways. Previous reports about the effects of livestock production on greenhouse gas emissions from the Food and Agriculture Organization (FAO) in 2006 showed the emissions to be far lower than what we now know. In 2010 UNESCO reported that "at least 51 percent of human-induced greenhouse gas emissions" are attributable to livestock production. This value is a significant upward revision from the FAO's 18 percent calculation,[61] representing an enormous shift in perspective and injecting impetus for innovations in our food supply.[62] Although the exact numbers may be up for debate, the problem is not.

The energy demands of livestock production are staggering, resulting in a serious loss of the calories and protein in cereals and legumes that could otherwise be used to meet human nutrition needs directly.[63] It takes thirty to forty times the fossil fuel energy to produce one pound of animal product than it does to produce just one pound of grain, but the energy requirements of producing animal products are just the tip of the wasteful iceberg with their real cost. When you factor in what is used to irrigate feed crops and pastures as well as the drinking water directly given to livestock, 50 percent of all the water used in the United States is given to the animals we eat.[64] Turning off the faucet while brushing our teeth will never have quite the impact on water conservation as simply choosing broccoli over beef, chickpeas over chicken.

Factory-farm animals are routinely administered "rapid grow" hormones.[65] This has become standard practice in the meat and dairy industries, where time is money, and we—right along with the animals—are the victims. Hormones are fed to beef cattle to make them ready for market all that much sooner, and bovine growth hormones are given to dairy cows to stimulate a higher level of IGF-1. These antibiotics and hormones are passed via the food chain right on to you in a supermarket smorgasbord of chemical-laden meat and milk.[66]

Increased public awareness of living conditions and treatment of livestock has also inspired the growing pull to plant-based eating. An important example in that realm is the plight of dairy cows. Cows, like all mammals, must be impregnated to produce milk, so they are kept in a constant unnatural cycle of impregnation, birth, and milking, with short rest between pregnancies. Most are kept indoors, with little to no access to outdoor concrete or dirt paddocks. Other problems include widespread infections and lameness,[67] surgical removal of their tails and dehorning (generally without painkillers), and separation of mother and baby. When a calf is born, he or she is rapidly removed from their mother to make the mother's milk available for dairy collection. Male offspring are then often raised for veal, while females become the next generation of dairy cows. Dairy cows usually meet their end at beef slaughterhouses, when, at two to five years of age, their milk production slows or they are too crippled or ill to continue in the dairy industry.[68]

Conditions for poultry are no better. Broiler chickens, bred and fed to rapidly grow from the size of your fist to the size of a soccer ball in about forty-five days, cannot bear the weight of their unnaturally large breasts and spend most of their time squatting.[69] Degenerative diseases and premature death abound. Over 90 percent of egg-laying hens spend their entire lives in battery cages—wire cubicles so small that not even one hen can extend her wings, let alone several more chickens in each cage—resulting in multiple health problems so common that the industry has a term for it: "cage fatigue."[70]

If you think switching to free-range and grass-fed meat and poultry is the answer, you'll have to think again: Apparently there aren't enough land and water resources to make this feel-good myth a viable option. And facility regulation does not inspire confidence.[71] Many of the problems of factory farms persist in smaller, free-range production.[72] And should you labor under the delusion that cows are building their bodies with plentiful green grass while contentedly roaming the lush green countryside, five minutes with Howard Lyman will enlighten you otherwise. Lyman is the conscience-driven soul who, after thirty-five years as a cattleman, was compelled to go public about the cattle industry's problematic practices in his book *Mad Cowboy*, seating him smack dab on Oprah's couch. His exposé of the problems with which ranches are riddled also landed him and Ms. Winfrey in court as they took turns on the hot seat of a defamation suit by the cattle industry. Says Lyman, "Evidently, telling the truth can get you into trouble." Apparently, according to Lyman, the famous marketing line "beef—it's what's for dinner" often applies to what the cows themselves are fed.[73] Conditions and treatment of livestock directly impact public and private health, and, along with depletion of natural resources, compounds an enormous ethical issue.[74]

Something's Fishy: Problems Presented by Fish— Whether Farmed or Fresh

For those who do cut out animal products, fish is often the last to go. A significant source of cholesterol and saturated fat, fish gets a lot of health hype for its omega-3 fatty acid content. But remember your sixth-grade science: Toxic elements such as mercury from our polluted waterways work their way up the food chain and become concentrated in the flesh and fats of fish. Farmed fish bring in a whole new set of complications. Not only are farmed fish fed meal made from smaller fish taken from contaminated areas, but they are also fed by-products from cows—another potential avenue for disease transmission through the food web.[75] Worldwide, supply for seafood like tuna and salmon is resulting in rapidly depleting populations of fish.[76] The problems associated with animal consumption—whether environmental, health, or ethical—are apparently associated with every farmed, harvested, or cultivated critter on our planet.

TAKE BACK YOUR PLATE

So how did we get into this mess hall mess? If it's all so simple, why didn't someone tell us? And why is there so much contrary information out there about good nutrition, keeping us in "what-should-I-eat!" whiplash? A little research reveals conflicts of interest all over even the U.S. Dietary Guidelines— guidelines that many a fine upstanding American citizen has come to accept as healthy mandate. The problem is, special interests have their fingerprints all over these guidelines—from subsidized food programs to sponsorship of nutrition education curriculums, brochures, and lesson plans implemented in our schools. Talk about moments of awakening. And apparently the USDA is obligated to promote dairy products, which, of course, shows up on the guidelines as well.[77,78]

Hope sprang with the publication of the 2010 U.S. Dietary Guidelines extolling the virtues of plant-based eating, stating, "Vegetarian-style eating patterns have been associated with improved health outcomes—lower levels of obesity, a reduced risk of cardiovascular disease, and lower total mortality." The guidelines then devote two full pages to plant-based nutrition, showing exactly how to easily pull together a healthy food plan. Uncle Sam's stamp of approval! While the USDA should be applauded for devoting space to plant-based eating, the guidelines need to take it several bites further. For even though they are clear about what we should be eating *more* of—fruits, vegetables, whole grains, and legumes—when it comes to what we should be eating *less* of, the guidelines use vague terms such as "cholesterol" and "saturated fat." Readers are left to their own devices to figure out where these come from. People don't eat cholesterol and saturated fat—they eat foods that contain them: meat and dairy products. Even Marion Nestle, professor in the department of nutrition at New York University, is quoted as saying that USDA Secretary Thomas Vilsack waffled when asked why the guidelines didn't clearly advise to reduce meat consumption. "This is no doubt to avoid the politically impossible 'eat less meat,'" Nestle responded.[79]

Where do you get the straight story? Interestingly, the Harvard School of Public Health—while supportive of the progressive elements of the 2010 USDA guidelines—takes issue with several of its details. Harvard suggests limits on animal products and getting our calcium from sources other than dairy, and has stated outright that the U.S. Dietary Guidelines are too lax on refined food.[80,81] Brilliant! Still, the U.S. government keeps pumping funds into research on heart disease and cancer while government subsidies push more meat, dairy, and refined foods onto our plates.

At the same time, a report on the healthfulness of our grocery purchases in light of compliance—or lack thereof—with the 2010 Guidelines stated, "Overall, consumers purchase too few fruits, vegetables, and whole grains and too many refined grains, fats, and sweets." In fact, the average consumer purchased barely half of the recommended whole plant foods.[82] Apparently, even the official proclamations guiding us to be healthy eaters are falling on dietary indiscriminate ears, easily influenced by convenience, marketing push, and taste-enhanced edibles.

But there's hope in high places. A 2009 advisory from the *American Journal of Clinical Nutrition* presented a report pointing to the importance of "various plant food–oriented recommendations . . . supported by literature evidence . . . that likely would improve health and the environment . . . oriented toward increased plant food consumption and some toward vegetarianism."[83] No doubt recommendations such as this exerted some degree of influence on the 2010 Guidelines. And encouraging words—directly from the 2015 U.S. Dietary Guidelines Advisory Committee notes—bring hope for weaving insight and vision into future dietary advisories by simply asking the question, "What is the relationship between population-level dietary patterns and long-term food sustainability and related food security?" Clearly, the environmental impact of food as played out in the "production, transport, retail, waste, etc." cycle, and the acknowledgment that viable dietary patterns exist that are "more plant-based," is on the table for committee discussion.[84]

The point I want to make is this. The wheels of government grind slowly, let alone those connected with healthy living. Thank goodness the government can to some extent protect us from a food contamination outbreak. But they can't protect us from the dietary damage we inflict upon ourselves. It is up to us as individuals to see the writing on the kitchen wall—and take charge of our own health by taking back our dinner plates. We cannot count on health care reform to do the work for us. Not when large-scale private interests still have such enormous influence over government policy on everything from pharmaceuticals to free school lunches. And not while health care is still perceived as disease management. Our goal should be health promotion and disease prevention. Making the paradigm shift from early detection to early prevention is going to need to be a grassroots movement. It starts with what you eat, which influences what your family eats, which then spreads to community and country. While genetics may load the launch pad, it is lifestyle that ignites the rockets. When you boil it down like this, the most immediate method of escaping these health-damaging—as well as conscience-com-promising and environmentally ravaging—problems, and enjoying radiant health, is clear: Eat more whole plant foods and less of everything else.

MODELS FOR CHANGE

Even as change from the top comes slowly, projects that support plant-based eating are being generated at the grassroots level and moving into encouraging expansion. Such take-back-your-plate initiatives inspire us to action. They provide us with models for change and the hope that healthier fare will become more available on a larger scale. Here are a couple of examples.

MUSE School: The Amis Cameron Connection

Suzy Amis Cameron and her husband, film director James Cameron, became environmental activists years ago. Inspired by such pro–plant-based diet works as *The China Study*, *Forks Over Knives*, *Food Choice and Sustainability*, and *Food Revolution*, they transitioned to a plant-based diet in 2012. Once they made the connection between personal dietary choices and the environment, they overhauled everything from the pantry to the family farm to eliminate animal products—overnight. "The connection between food and the environment has been a major eye-opener," says Suzy. "Our family is benefiting greatly from eating plant-based—but the environmental piece has become our primary focus."[85]

A natural outcome of their interest was the creation of the environmentally focused MUSE School, located in Southern California. Founded by Suzy and her sister Rebecca Amis in 2006, MUSE was created "to inspire and prepare young people to live consciously with themselves, one another, and the planet." At MUSE, conscious living now means being conscious right down to what they eat in the school dining room.

At MUSE, students and staff are growing fresh fruits and vegetables as they increase the presence of plants on their plate. "We are gradually moving toward a 100 percent plant-based menu—because we do call ourselves an environmental school," Suzy says. "By fall 2015, we will be all plant-based."[86] And the Amis-Cameron team isn't stopping there. They are planning a global campaign to persuade people to move toward a plant-only diet in order to sharply reduce global carbon emissions and improve their health.

Hampton Creek

Challenging the multibillion-dollar chicken egg industry, Hampton Creek, a northern California technology company pioneering in food, is screening plants for their functional capability in food products. Plants like the Canadian yellow pea are able to replace the function of a chicken's egg in foods like mayonnaise and cookie dough—even scrambled eggs. Bill Gates—along with several other investors, to the tune of some $30 million—has leaned substantial financial weight into Hampton Creek's mission to make the food system better, by making the healthier options the more affordable ones.[87] "Using plants is better because they are more sustainable, healthy, easy to transport, affordable, and efficient—and without the environmental externalities," says founder Josh Tetrick.[88] A personal tour and taste test at the Hampton Creek kitchen with Tetrick proved the gustatory worthiness and market viability of their products—underscored now by the Hampton Creek shelf presence at Safeway, Costco, Whole Foods Market, Target, Amazon, and Walmart, as well as its growing use in industrial food products from companies such as General Mills and Ikea. Taking the eggs out of mayonnaise, cookies, and scrambled eggs and replacing them with plant ingredients is proving to be more sustainable and less costly—good news for discriminate and budget-minded consumers.

• • •

News and research urging the shift to a plant-based diet continue to multiply. Perhaps some of the incentives touched upon here have given you a fresh connection or cause for commitment, compelling you forward on the plant-based journey. Whether your reasons are singular or many, your desired changes small or sweeping, it's time to make your ideals resonate on your plate.

This transition—shifting to a plant-based lifestyle—is for each of us a personal journey. It's a journey I've traveled now for over four decades. Perhaps telling you a little about my own is a good place to go next.

PLANT-BASED JOURNEY RESOURCES

To download a rich reserve of lists and resources—everything from scientific research to support systems, access to endless plant-centered recipes, food prep tips, and books that educate and inspire—go to www.theplantbasedjourney. com and navigate to Resources.

CHAPTER 2
My Plant-Based Journey

There is a snapshot of me at four years of age, standing next to a big slab of meat roasting on a barbecue. The look on my face is clearly disgruntled, no doubt about something entirely unrelated to what is sizzling on the spit next to me. Yet considering my longtime passion for plant-based anything, it makes for an interesting photograph.

Another picture taken of me as a pudgy toddler points to my genetic predisposition to easily gain—and have difficulty shaking—excess weight. A look back through the family photo album reveals a long line of relatives burdened with excess avoirdupois. Being a professional health and fitness educator didn't make the years of struggle with my weight any easier.

POINTS, PORTIONS, DIET PRISON, AND PERSONALLY HITTING BOTTOM

Perhaps the lowest point in my complex, beleaguered quest for the magic weight loss bullet came several decades into the melee. I had white-knuckled my way through several days of a popular diet—you'd recognize the name, as it is synonymous with "low carb"—in an effort to force the fat off. Low-carb diets can be vege-tized, and it is possible—though difficult—to pull them off. As an egg-free vegetarian, following this diet meant consuming endless chunks of cheese—which I was eating at the time—and blocks of tofu. My craving for carbohydrates became so extreme that I found myself rifling through the recipe section of the diet book for something sweet—anything sweet—that I could eat without blasting through my meager carbohydrate allotment for the day. I found a recipe for fudge, but there was one problem. As it could contain no ingredients with more than a whisper of carbohydrate, guess what comprised the foundation of the recipe? In addition to the cocoa, the main ingredient was paraffin. That's right. The petroleum-based diet. I'd never thought to stock my pantry with paraffin. But there was no stopping me now. I rushed out and bought paraffin, melted it down, made the fudge, and clawed my way through the pan, polishing off the entire batch. I may have had fossil fuel dribbling down my chin, but I didn't overshoot my carbs. I still have the remainder of the block of paraffin in the back of my pantry. I use it to wax the tracks on our sliding doors.

Though this certainly makes an interesting story, my point is this. Why was I so helpless at sticking with a weight loss food plan for more than a few days at a time before my hunger drive overcame my best intentions to lose a few pounds? Although I was certain it was true at the time, I've since learned that I wasn't a hopeless food addict. I was just hungry.

MY "WHY"

When I started on the plant-based journey over four decades ago, my reasons then were just as they are now. Back then, I was prompted by 1) my health and weight, and 2) the Trojan horse of troubles inherent in animal product production, including 3) environmental issues. The quest for the first has been happily resolved and keeps me enthusiastically on the plant-based path. The other two reasons are, sadly, not only still alive and kicking today, but they have also become even more compelling. The implications of what we choose to eat, as underscored in chapter 1, have become ever more profound.

In spite of the snapshot of me next to the roast on the barbecue, I do give credit to my parents for instilling in me early on the importance of healthy eating and exercise. Mom wouldn't be caught red-handed with doughnuts or their junk food relatives in the house—except on rare occasions when Dad's renowned sweet tooth prevailed. Some of my earliest memories of going to the market with Mom were ventures to the health food store for sugar-free whatever. Dad's green thumb and my parents' passion for home-grown anything delivered to our family a huge fruit and vegetable garden. They grew everything from eggplant to towering rows of boysenberries. Anything that couldn't be consumed fresh was frozen and stored in our freezer or dried on the roof in the sun. Summers were filled with camping excursions and outdoor adventures. The foundation for good eating and active living was laid early on.

I ventured into eating plant-based long before the term was coined. Back then it was simply vegetarian with a few variations on the theme. When I undertook the study of yoga, I learned about vegetarianism—a natural extension. In college I progressed to teaching yoga classes, and—along with my soon-to-be-husband, Greg—eating a vegetarian diet. My reasons today for this choice were already issues on the table back then. I still have an early booklet on vegetarianism, "Meat on the Menu: Who Needs It?" dated 1973. To be honest, all the while I was secretly hoping that going veg would once and for all end my struggle with weight. Yet as I soon learned, vegetarian isn't synonymous with skinny, and doesn't necessarily mean healthy.

Our eating style was challenged two years in when, as newlyweds, we signed on for the Peace Corps. We envisioned serving in Southeast Asia, where, among other reasons, we knew it would probably be fairly easy to find plenty of vegetarian-friendly fare. Imagine our befuddlement when we were assigned to Afghanistan. Keep in mind this was before any of us knew where Afghanistan was. Our vision of strumming guitars, singing with children, and changing lives in a lush, green, veg-friendly locale was abruptly replaced by head-to-toe coverage in clothing and a thick layer of dust in sunbaked downtown Kabul, where we were first stationed to learn Pashtu in language class. Though our Afghan adventure is an entire story in and of itself, for the food part, we found ourselves in the land of the meat kabob. Bowls of soup floated an inch-thick layer of sheep fat on top. And don't dare send it back without risk of highly offending the host, a huge taboo as international ambassadors. We were hard-pressed to find food we could eat. The French Bakery in Kabul stocked yogurt—dairy was still on the menu at the time. If it weren't for that and Aziz' Ice Cream Parlor—which we frequented until we discovered it was ground zero for a local outbreak of tuberculosis—eating vegetarian while living in the training compound would have, on the face of it, seemed impossible. Undaunted, we pulled together a meal plan with rice, crisp flat bread pried from the walls of wood-burning ovens, vegetables, and intermittent boosts from the bakery—a testament to what can be done in plant-perplexing situations.

Within a few years, our passion for wildlife and the environment started taking us all over the world volunteering as field biologists. It granted us exotic experiences such as protecting sea turtles on the beaches in Costa Rica and Mexico, participating in rain forest preservation projects in Ecuador and Belize, and monitoring albatross nests on Midway Island. These experiences cemented our commitment to eating low on the food chain. Seeing firsthand the destruction to the environment and wildlife caused by humankind's insatiable desire to exploit the landscape for animal products reinforced our lifestyle choices. It deeply informed our work as environmental educators, and underscored the value of thinking outside yourself for making meaningful change. These experiences stressed how simple it is to make a difference in this one way—by what we put on our plate.

My last animal product dietary holdout was dairy. I had known from early on about the multiple problems inherent in the dairy industry, but I was only sporadically successful at cutting their products out of my diet. Yet the case against consumption of dairy products only compounded over the years. For a long time I had compartmentalized the problem in my head. Compartmentalization can be a useful tool when you can't change the circumstances. But when it comes to taking an inappropriate food off your plate, it's a whole other story. You can change the circumstances. You come to understand that it now becomes a matter of confronting long-seated gustatory preferences—and, in this case, the dairy industry whitewash that has convinced us that if we aren't drinking two glasses of milk a day our bodies will collapse in a heap of shattered bones. The grip of dairy products can be insidious—their consumption triggers a highly pleasurable biochemical response, no doubt the reason that many people find cheese one of the hardest animal products to forgo.[1] Finally, after a short series of events several years ago—well into my plant-based journey—I dropped dairy products.

Five events converged to inspire me to eat dairy-free, and they plugged into all of my reasons for living plant-based. For one, I attended a daylong physician's seminar that graphically underscored the human health problems correlated with dairy product consumption. Granted, I'd heard much of this before. But evidence continues to mount, and this added to the monumental documentation that dairy products do not do a body good—in fact, they do more harm than I'd thought. This started to chip away at my compartmentalization. Second, I also realized that eating dairy was not helping me with my weight problem. Third, the accurately descriptive, paradigm-shifting term "animals and their secretions" snapped me to attention. Fourth, the environmental degradation that results from animal agriculture—including dairy—was clearly not going away but rather growing in magnitude. Finally, video footage of the handling of dairy cows edified the switch.[2] To this day, when I see a carton of milk, it is those cows that I see.

Some of the obvious and immediate rewards from dropping dairy products were easier weight management, no more ear infections—which had plagued me for years—and the clarity and confidence that come when you live more in alignment with your ideals.

As the decades have advanced since I first pushed meat off my plate, the marketplace has become more and more plant-friendly, making it easy to go almost anywhere in the world and find good things to eat—a far cry from the days when restaurant waitstaff would reply to our questions about the menu with "vege-what?" The same is true internationally. Whether in Italy, Switzerland, Mexico, Honduras, the Philippines, Indonesia, Palau, Africa, Borneo, or the Dutch Antilles, I've found it's usually easy to ask for what I want and get it.

With increased availability of plant-based options, we have an instant leg up on the journey. To further close the gap between your current dietary practices and your aspirations, you will need an action plan. The doctors, research scientists, and dietitians give us the essential raw materials that are the foundation of plant-based living. Connecting it all with your reality? That is where I come in. It took me trial, error, and a long trail of tears to figure out how to realize my ideal weight—finally found in this simple, healthy, satisfying, research-driven, personally resonant, and lasting way. I've made all the mistakes so you don't have to. I share every bit of it with you via the proven solutions, strategies, and action steps in this book.

SECTION 2

SCOUT

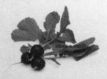

Getting Ready and Setting the Stage for Success

CHAPTER 3
The Plant-Based Plate

Once you've discovered your "why" for eating plant-based, the next step is to transition into actual plant-based eating. What do you eat when following a plant-based diet? What do you not eat? When it comes to making changes with what's on your plate, meal plans and recipes point out the possibilities. Yet they can still leave you with questions. What does *real* dining—meal by meal—on a whole food, plant-based diet look like? And how do you get there from where you are? It's time to answer all those important, juicy questions about how to simply get started. The Scout reconnaissance expedition is under way.

In this chapter we'll shine a spotlight on what plant-based means, discovering which foods you'll be moving more of *onto* your plate and which you'll be crowding *off* of your plate. To give you an example of what day-to-day eating plant-based might look like, I've also included a personal food journal. Most of all, I want to show you how simple and fun it is to do this. Meanwhile, you get to enjoy the many tasty, slimming, and energizing benefits of plant-based eating—every step of the way.

WHAT IS PLANT-BASED?

Plant-based literally means that the great majority of energy—you might call it calories—that you eat come from plants, and foods made from them. If in your mind's eye when you think "plants" you envision flowering gardens and green leaves, pull back until that picture expands to include apples, potatoes, and everything else that photosynthesizes. Whole foods are also important to discuss when talking about a healthy plant-based diet, because the focus of studies documenting the health-promoting power of plant-based eating is based upon primarily plant foods in their whole, unrefined form. Discouraged are meats, dairy products, eggs, highly refined carbohydrates, and the added fats used—more often than not—in making convenience foods.[1] Being a "whole food" means that a plant food has all of its original parts in place, and is minimally altered from its original form. For our purposes, we'll use the term "plant-based" to refer to these foods for the most part, to avoid the important yet cumbersome "whole food, plant-based." This eating approach is rich in all the nutrition you need to thrive with optimal health and to easily reach—and maintain—your ideal weight.

As you get started eating plant-based, rather than worry about getting in X number of servings from any particular plant food group each day, it's more important that you delight in your meals, that your food tastes really good, and that you feel satisfied. You can think about food as being in three categories: 1) plant-based, 2) animal-based, and 3) refined/processed.[2] As long as you're eating as much as you can from the first category—plant-based foods—while minimizing or eliminating the other two, you'll be well on your way.

Rather than obtaining nutrients from animal products—where you might be used to getting them—you'll be getting them directly from where the animals got them in the first place: plants! By essentially bypassing the middleman, you'll get all the goodies—vitamins, minerals, phytonutrition, fiber, protein, fats, and carbohydrates—directly from the plant world, without the cholesterol, saturated fat, bioaccumulated toxins, and other problems associated with animal products.

So, is that all you really need to know? Can't this section just end here? Yes and no. There can be a learning curve to getting started. Some people, in their earnestness to "get it right," become easily distracted, lost in the details of eating certain foods to the exclusion of others in a search for some plant-based offshoot of a dietary magic bullet. Some try to eat mostly vegetables, yet remain hungry and calorie deprived because they aren't eating sufficiently of more robust choices, such as the starches and beans. Or they're trying to eat all raw salads and can't find enough hours in the day to chew, keeping satisfaction elusive. These are common pitfalls that can actually prevent you from enjoying the plant-based approach at the outset, which is why I mention them here. Once you realize that the comfort foods you already enjoy—blueberry pancakes, bean burritos, chili with corn bread—should take up generous real estate on your plate, it sheds a whole new, exciting light on the meaning of plant-based.

The Plant-Based Plate and the Five Food Groups

Nonstarchy vegetables, "starchies" (starchy vegetables and whole grains), beans and legumes, fruits, and nuts and seeds fill the Plant-Based Plate. Below, you'll find lists with just some of the options for plant-based foods. You'll also find serving suggestions, included not to encourage dietary dogmatism but because one of the challenges of going plant-based is making sure that you eat *enough*. This is a detail of transition that I find needs addressing more often than not. Whole plant foods take up a lot more space on your plate than do animal products and processed foods. That means you get to eat—and must eat—greater quantities than what you might be accustomed to eating. Eat enough servings to satisfy your hunger.

Take a look at these five food groups, pick out the types of food you already like, and start eating more of them. The idea is to eat abundantly of whole plant foods, and enjoy what you eat, while at the same time crowding out animal products and refined foods.

Plant-Based Food Group	Examples	Suggested Servings
Nonstarchy Vegetables With only trace amounts of starch in them, these are high in water and less energy dense than starchy vegetables.	Artichokes, arugula, asparagus, basil, bok choy, broccoli, Brussels sprouts, cabbage, cauliflower, celery, cucumber, eggplant, green beans, green onion, mushrooms, okra, parsley, peppers, zucchini, and a long list of leafy greens, including spinach, romaine, Swiss chard, collard greens, kale, lettuce, mustard greens, and rhubarb	Unlimited, yet aim for a minimum of seven servings a day, including at least two servings of leafy greens. **One serving:** 1 cup raw; ½ cup cooked

Plant-Based Food Group	Examples	Suggested Servings
Starchies Whole grains and starchy vegetables make up the "starchies" category. They have similar properties yet important differences, so you'll want to include plenty of servings from each. Along with beans and legumes, these robust, satisfying, nutrition-packed gems take center stage on your plate. Together they are key to satiety and easy weight management.	**Starchy vegetables and tubers:** butternut, acorn, and other hearty squashes, potatoes, sweet potatoes, yams, beets, carrots, corn, and peas **Whole grains:** amaranth, barley, buckwheat, corn, kamut, millet, oats, quinoa, rye, rice, spelt, wheat; cracked grains such as bulgur and other forms of whole grains (whole grain flours, whole wheat couscous, polenta, whole grain pasta, whole grain tortillas or sandwich wraps, whole wheat breads and buns, and baked tortilla chips without added oils)	Seven to twelve or more servings a day as energy needs demand. **One serving:** ½ cup cooked; 1 slice bread or tortilla
Beans and Legumes Technically qualifying as a starch, beans and legumes are highlighted separately here to underscore their unique value and the tremendous variety the plant world delivers.	Adzuki beans, black beans, black-eyed peas, cannellini beans, chickpeas (garbanzo beans), kidney beans, lentils, lima beans, peanuts, split peas, pinto beans, white beans, soybeans/edamame, tofu, and tempeh	Aim for two to four servings a day. **One serving:** ½ cup cooked
Fruits Enjoy every day, staying mindful of the primary role of starchies and vegetables.	Apples, bananas, berries, cherries, grapes, grapefruit, kiwi, lemons, mangoes, oranges, papaya, pears, peaches, pomegranates, mandarins, and melons	Two to four servings a day. **One serving:** 1 piece or about ½ cup
Nuts, Seeds, and Other High-Fat Plant Foods Providing important nutrition, nuts and seeds are also very energy dense. This means that bite for bite you consume more calories than any other whole plant food. Eat sparingly if you are seeking to lose weight, more if you want to gain or are extremely active and need the extra calories to keep up with energy demands.	**Nuts and seeds:** almonds, cashews, coconut, hazelnuts, peanuts (officially a legume), pecans, pine nuts, pistachios, walnuts, flaxseeds, sesame seeds, sunflower seeds, and nut and seed butters and flours **Other high-fat plant foods:** avocados and olives	Up to one or more servings per day, as compatible with your health, weight, and activity level. **One serving:** 1 ounce of nuts or 1–2 tablespoons seeds; 2 tablespoons nut butter; ¼ avocado; 3–5 olives

Crowd These Off of Your Plate

While staying focused on the new eating options that have just opened up, these are the items to start crowding off of your plate—while simultaneously upping the presence of whole plant foods.

Category	Why You Should Eat Less
Animal products: meat, fish, poultry, dairy, and eggs	Consuming these introduces harmful elements into your body, such as increased animal protein, cholesterol, saturated fat, and chemicals that have bioaccumulated in animal tissues. This not only rapidly taxes your body, but it also displaces the nutrition essentials supplied by plant foods.
Highly refined processed products: products made with refined white flour, sugar, fats, and oils such as pastries, cookies, cakes, and expelled vegetables oils	Sweets and pastries are fleeced of their original fiber, vitamins, minerals, and phytochemicals, and deliver a surge of sugar and fat to your body. This can heighten your risk for disease and weight gain. The same goes for vegetable oils—at 120 calories per tablespoon the most calorie-concentrated edible there is.

THE PLANT-BASED JOURNAL

To give you a better idea of how these eating guidelines might play out in practice, I've provided a food journal below, detailing my typical meals over the course of a week. This peek at my plate will give you an idea of the possibilities, and what it might look like for *you* eating plant-based—so you can say, "I can do that!" It is by no means a prescriptive, or an exact outline that you should follow bite-for-bite. The danger with providing a meals model is that you may feel compelled to follow it exactly. This is not the intention—yet it can give you a guide from which to create your *own* Plant-Based Plate. At the same time, you are welcome to try out my food choices. It might just help you find your own style.

Though specifics vary according to personal preferences, you will find the plant-based basics here. Remember, at this stage you are gathering information. Let it liberate you and open the door to new options. Let it show you how much you actually get to eat—and how fun and simple this whole plant-based thing is. Experiment!

LEAFY GREENS

If you are familiar with lettuce, spinach, or cabbage, then you are already acquainted with leafy greens. These include all lettuce varieties, kale, collards, turnip greens, beet greens, and chard, for starters. Leafy greens are a rich source of nutrients such as calcium, iron, protein, fiber, and folate—the word "folate" is derived from the word "foliage." You'll even find omega-3 fatty acids in those leaves, too.

And you needn't consume massive amounts to take advantage of the benefits. Start with a couple of servings a day and work your way up. That's easy to achieve with, for example, a mixed green salad and bowl of steamed spinach.

Seven-Day Plant-Based Journal

Day 1	Meal	Notes
6:45 A.M.	Oatmeal, topped with raisins, banana slices, a big scoop of blueberries, and a tablespoon of ground flaxseed	Oatmeal is a frequent and favorite breakfast choice. Sometimes it is old-fashioned rolled oats, sometimes steel-cut oats, sometimes in the form of muesli, and sometimes a big bowl of whole oats, cooked by themselves or with other grains. Often I'll sprinkle on chopped walnuts or other nuts or seeds. For fruit, I pick from what is in season that I have on hand. I always make sure I have blueberries or mixed berries frozen as backup—they're always in season in my freezer!
11:45 A.M.	Large bowl of Simple Vegetable Soup Hummus, tomato, avocado, and onion sandwich on whole grain bread	One of the easiest, most satisfying ways to increase your vegetable count is through soup. I cook a large quantity to last a few days. As an added bonus, I often toss in several handfuls of greens such as baby kale to further "plantify" the meal—they cook quickly in the heat of the soup. My sandwich is bursting with a favorite filling—hummus—which lends itself to endless variations on a theme.
5:00 P.M.	Large baby spinach and romaine salad Big bowl of Game-Changer Chili Country Comfort Corn Bread	A couple of times a week I cook a large batch of beans—black, kidney, pinto—which I keep on hand for adding to soups, salads, and chili such as I made for tonight's dinner. I also keep an inventory of canned beans handy in the pantry for last-minute food prep.

Day 2	Meal	Notes
7:00 A.M.	Steamy bowl of brown rice cream with a small amount of raisins, a chopped apple, and a dab of peanut butter stirred in, topped with a splash of plant milk	One of my favorite combinations is rice cream, raisins, and peanut butter. Together these make breakfast an absolute dessert—and why not? I also love the crunch of fresh chopped apple for texture.
12:00 P.M.	Large salad of grated cabbage and carrots topped with cold cooked green peas, a big scoop of chickpeas, sweet balsamic vinegar as dressing, all topped with a couple of tablespoons of Red Star nutritional yeast and a tablespoon of lightly toasted sunflower seeds	There's nothing like a food processor to make big salads fast and easy. Sometimes I will shred an entire head of cabbage and put it in a quart-size container in the refrigerator. I'll do the same with carrots. This way for two to three days all I need to do is slide those containers out of the fridge and voilà—instant salad. My favorite go-to dressing is very easy—which it needs to be, as I want it ready quick. I simply drizzle the salad with a good aged balsamic vinegar or a squeeze of lemon or lime juice. Often I'll use Sweet and Sour Dressing. Another good option is hummus thinned with brown rice vinegar, or lime juice blended with dates, dill, and tahini, or sesame butter. Adding seeds, like sunflower seeds, lends a rich flavor when combined with the dressing.
5:00 P.M.	Indian Plant Burger on a sprouted whole grain bun with sweet onion, tomato, and mango chutney Big heap of steamed green beans	I made a large double batch of the burgers to keep on hand in the fridge for meals in the days ahead.

Day 3	Meal	Notes
7:00 A.M.	Mandarin oranges Pumpkin Muffins	Although I usually opt for a bowl of whole grains for breakfast, I'll sometimes make pancakes, waffles, or muffins.
12:00 P.M.	Avocado and tomato sandwich with onion and mustard on whole grain bread Large salad with grated cabbage, carrot, and sweet balsamic vinegar and lemon as dressing	With the containers of shredded carrots and cabbage in the fridge, I am all set with everything needed to make a robust salad in less than 2 minutes.

5:00 P.M.	Buddha Bowl: baby spinach, black rice, steamed broccoli florets, red bell pepper, and Indian Plant Burger croquettes, with Tahini-Lemon Sauce	Buddha Bowls are among the simplest, quickest, and most pleasing meals to make. I started with a couple of handfuls of raw spinach in the bottom of large, wide pasta bowls, perfect for this purpose. On top of the spinach I heaped steaming black rice, then scattered the broccoli and a few thin slices of the fresh red pepper over the top. I cut two Indian Plant Burgers left over from yesterday into six bite-size pieces each, and quickly dry-roasted to crisp in a nonstick pan—my "croquettes"—placed those on top, and drizzled the sauce lightly over all.

Day 4	Meal	Notes
7:15 A.M.	Mandarin orange Steel-cut oats with a scoop of Sweet Bean Cream folded in and topped with one chopped apple, a tablespoon of ground flaxseed, and a splash of plant milk	The staying power that beans give you is so profound that I was determined to find a way to make them part of breakfast. I hit the nail on the head with Sweet Bean Cream. A scoop of this folded into hot grains adds a fluffy sweetness that brings all the goodness of the beans along with it. It's also a great topper for toast, muffins, and pancakes.
12:00 P.M.	Hummus, tomato, onion, and avocado on whole grain bread Large salad of grated cabbage, carrot, chopped parsley, raisins, and sweet balsamic vinegar as dressing	The food processor makes it easy to prepare big batches of substantial, zesty hummus that works perfectly as either a full sandwich filling, to moisten the bread, or to simply scoop into the center of a large salad.
5:30 P.M.	Bowl of sugar snap peas Large scoop of Golden Turmeric Rice topped with baked tofu chunks A heap of steamed Brussels sprouts lightly drizzled with Sweet and Sour Dressing	The sugar snap peas I munched on while doing the simple steps of preparation for this meal. This way I get the benefit of additional vegetables without going through the motions of actually preparing a salad—think outside the salad bowl! The rice was loaded into the rice cooker 45 minutes earlier, so it would be ready on time. The Brussels sprouts are a fast preparation—simply trim off the bottoms, chop the larger ones in half, and pressure cook for 5–7 minutes, depending on their size. I chunked some seasoned, baked tofu (ready-made at many markets) and used it to decorate the scoops of rice on our plates.

Day 5	Meal	Notes
6:30 A.M.	Sliced navel orange A couple slices of sprouted whole grain raisin toast with almond butter and jam	With an early morning departure for a day on the road, it was up and out the door early. Whole grain toast with a thin coating of nut butter did the trick.
11:15 A.M.	Giant carrot and chunk of cabbage Large bowl of vegetable soup: onion, mushrooms, thinly sliced Brussels sprouts, chunks of baked potato, some kidney beans, and a handful of baby kale stirred in at the last minute	While preparing a big pot of soup for lunch—with the idea of making plenty for the next few days—I did something I often do and enjoyed a carrot and a chunk of cabbage, upping my vegetable count for the day.
5:30 P.M.	Super-size spinach salad Baked potato, sliced and heated on nonstick stove top Mixed sweet corn and vegetables	Even though lunch was early, it was so robust it kept me energized well into the afternoon. I had planned on doing more with the big batch of baked potatoes I had cooked a couple of days before, but when I went to get dinner going, there weren't as many potatoes as I had planned for. This called for last-minute dinner thinking—an easy need met by keeping a veggie stash in the freezer. I grabbed a bag of frozen corn and frozen mixed vegetables, emptied them side by side into a glass dish, popped on the lid, and cooked them for 6 minutes in the microwave. Dinner was a smash with the dark green salad, the brilliant corn and mixed veggies, and sliced crispy potatoes on the side, all seasoned with some sweet vinegar and a splash of red ketchup on the potatoes. It really is that easy to make a meal.

Day 6	Meal	Notes
7:00 A.M.	Bowl of mixed oatmeal and polenta with a chopped large pear, sprinkling of chopped walnuts, dried apricots, and a splash of soy milk	The sweetness of corn shines through today's morning oatmeal via the polenta.
12:15 P.M.	Massaged kale salad with grated carrots, torn baby spinach, and cooked yam cut into chunks, topped with balsamic vinegar and lemon juice Corn tortillas with black beans and salsa	Massaged kale sounds exotic and its taste is also extraordinary—yet it is deceptively easy to make. I simply emptied a bag of torn kale from the supermarket into a bowl, drizzled with a good vinegar and the juice from a wedge of lemon, and kneaded the bright green pile for barely 30 seconds. This process softens the fibers of the kale and turns it a brilliant velvet green. This salad was a feast for the eyes and one of the most satisfying lunch bowls in recent memory. I spooned hot black beans onto warmed corn tortillas, then spooned on heaps of mild salsa and served them as roll-ups to complete the meal.
6:00 P.M.	Big serving of Black Bean Polenta Pie Large romaine salad with Sweet and Sour Dressing	For the most part I shy away from recipes in preference of just throwing something simple together. Yet Black Bean Polenta Pie is worth the effort—a crowd-pleaser, husband-pleaser, and kid-pleaser too.

Day 7	Meal	Notes
7:00 A.M.	Whole Grain Breakfast Template with a scoop of Sweet Bean Cream, kiwi and banana slices, a tablespoon of ground flaxseed, and a splash of almond milk	Mixing and matching whole grains that haven't been cracked or rolled delivers a breakfast with a wonderful, unique texture. A favorite combination is oat groats and wheat berries.
10:00 A.M.	Baked sweet potato, one large carrot	Last night I had pressure-cooked a heap of red potatoes, yellow potatoes, and sweet potatoes and yams, giving me a nice bowl of leftovers to select from. And yes, taters at ten are a fresh and satisfying way to fuel up midmorning if you need it.
12:00 P.M.	Large salad containing grated carrots, cabbage, and English peas A heaping scoop of Golden Turmeric Rice Serving of black beans on the side	Left over from the other night's dinner, Golden Turmeric Rice is a fragrant family favorite—colorful, chewy, and nutty with the addition of chickpeas—with just the right amount of sweet from the raisins.

5:30 P.M.	Large romaine lettuce salad with white balsamic vinegar Mixed peas and corn, topped with cubes of baked, seasoned cubed tofu	The beans, rice, and salad for lunch piggybacked on the potatoes midmorning, and ferried me well through the day. When hunger hit early evening it was easy to pull together a simple dinner by opening a bag of romaine lettuce, quickly cooking some peas and corn pulled from the freezer, and tossing a few bites of tofu on top.
7:30 P.M.	Medium-size bowl of air-popped popcorn	I top my popcorn with a fresh grind of garlic salt for a savory snack, or cinnamon for sweet!

As you can see, my meals follow a pattern. Breakfast is usually whole grains with fruit. Lunch? A large bowl of hearty salad or soup with, quite often, a sandwich. For dinner, I'll select a starchy vegetable or whole grain and nonstarchy vegetables, steamed, pressure-cooked, or prepared Savory Vegetables style—often served with a light sauce or vinaigrette, more salad, and usually beans or legumes. Sometimes these ingredients find their way into more structured recipes, several of which I've provided for you in chapters 8 and 14. Patterns prevail, yet deviations are completely normal. I maximize whole and minimally processed foods. I don't eat any animal products. And I don't eat anything I don't like.

These meals are typical, yet not necessarily the rule. When I'm south of the border, nothing suits me better than beans, corn tortillas, and salsa with a side of mango and papaya for breakfast. I've had miso soup with vegetables and noodles for breakfast in the Pacific Islands, and black beans and rice for the first meal of the day in Costa Rica. Plant-centered plates can vary greatly, depending on individual tastes, preferences, food sensitivities, or the nuances of travel. That's half the fun. For example, my friend Alicia dines early on a mountain of steamed greens, sometimes adding a flavored vinegar or nutty dressing, with a sweet potato or whole grains and fruit on the side. Another friend, Colleen, thrives on a tall green smoothie of blended spinach and other leafy greens, and fresh fruits with chia seeds stirred in. My friend Rick favors scrambled tofu with whole wheat toast and sliced tomatoes. The important rule here is that plants rule.

CARBS REKINDLED: COMFORT FOODS TAKE CENTER STAGE

Fluffy mashed potatoes with gravy, plump golden yams bursting at the seams, steamy heaps of fragrant rice, piles of pasta, filling bowls of chili with sweet corn bread, and glistening golden corn on the cob. If these comfort foods sound good to you, it's because it's your birthright. That's right, it's in your DNA. With the aid of molecular genetics, research confirms that humans, due to the proliferation of genes for producing amylase—the enzyme that starts the digestion of starch—are marvelously equipped to digest starches for energy and thrive on starch as found in whole grains and starchy vegetables.[3] You knew it! Longtime carbophobic[4] holdouts—I used to be one of them—take note. This is a good time to point out that all carbohydrates are not created equal. The low-carb media frenzy we've had to endure as a by-product of high-protein diet marketing has misled us by lumping all carbohydrates together—the health-compromising highly refined carbohydrates right in there with the health-building whole plant variety. Take, for example, those popular potato chips that come stacked in a can. Only faintly reminiscent of potatoes, these chips are formed from a slurry of highly refined potato flour, corn flour, wheat starch, and rice flour together with fat and emulsifier, salt and seasonings, and then pressed into shape. Potato content—and denatured at that, with barely any vestiges of fiber or other important nutrition real potatoes champion—is only about 42 percent.[5] So they aren't really potatoes at all. In contrast, a potato baked whole or sliced and cooked is a whole food complete with fiber, micronutrients, and complex phytonutrition.

THE BRIGHTER THE BETTER!

Phytonutrients, also known as phytochemicals—*phyto* literally translates from the Greek word for "plant"—are bioactive chemical compounds found in plants. They are not categorized as vitamins or minerals, yet are considered to be beneficial to human health and enhance immune function.

Antioxidants buffer plant tissue from the stresses of photosynthesis, the process by which plants make food. Plants practice damage control by assembling antioxidants that also help protect plants from germs, fungi, bugs, and other threats. The same protection from oxidation that these molecules provide for plants, they bestow on us. Health protective and disease preventive, they function to detoxify damage in your body resulting from normal metabolic processes and environmental stresses such as air pollution. There are thousands of known antioxidants, and they are believed to work most effectively in combination with one another, just as they are found naturally occurring in whole plant foods. These antioxidants are what give plants their brilliant color—the properties they provide us with when we eat plants is no doubt the reason their color has such universal appeal for the human eye.

When delivered in the complete package as nature intended, whole starchy carbohydrate foods, such as potatoes, whole grains, yams, and squashes, come with fiber, antioxidants, protein, and fats. They are a perfect match for our bodies. It's only when we mess with carbohydrates by hacking them to bits—through refining them, separating out key nutritional elements, and pulling out their parts—that we can get into trouble with carbs.

OCCASIONAL OTHERS

We seem to have a love/hate relationship with change, for as excited as we are about the good things that will come to pass as we shift to occupying our plates with plants, we can also be reluctant to let the less desirables go. Even though you have voted these edibles off the island, there can be a resulting sense of loss. These are natural and normal red flags of change, and can show up as thoughts such as, "I can never have X again!"

PLANT PERFECT?

Perfection? I do not aspire to eat "plant-perfect," make a perfect soufflé, set the perfect table, or do anything else perfectly, other than be perfectly happy. As a matter of fact, one of my favorite phrases is "perfect enough," which I picked up while traveling on the small island of Dominica. Here, delivery of farm food to your door can be intermittent, electric power iffy, and other services hit or miss. At first, our hostess asked us about our ease with this arrangement, aka island "normal." We responded with "Of course! No problem!" to which she replied, "Oh good. We have a phrase here on the island: Perfect enough."

So don't look at it that way. I don't. If you were to tell me I could never have another glass of champagne or piece of birthday cake, well, just take me out now. I'll tell you what I do instead. I employ a distinct tactic that I call "occasional others." This means planning desserts or special dinners with richer fare than usual. I stay away from animal products, but I'll occasionally nudge the line into richer plant fare. When you give yourself permission to intermittently indulge like this, you disarm the internal rebel by making it your friend. I implement this strategy during the holidays, too, and have devised a very successful system of selecting specific events at which I will indulge. This prevents the unconscious topple that can start at Halloween, precipitating a processed foods sleigh ride all the way through Thanksgiving and into the New Year. When I *plan* to enjoy that Thanksgiving nut roast, or the cashew chocolate mousse pie at Christmas—richer food than I would usually find on my plate on a typical day—it satisfies the mind and makes it easy to eat well day in and day out.

There are some individuals who, whether due to acute health problems or fear of food itself, swear by drawing a line in the sand between themselves and any dietary leniency. For some this can be a workable approach. For others it builds more tension in a brittle black-or-white thinking wall that easily snaps, leaving you vulnerable to an eat-everything-in-sight ambush. Dietary rigidity can amplify dietary disinhibition, veering you even further off course.[6] Perhaps you know the feeling. How often can you indulge in the occasional other? Just as in transition styles, each person must find what works best for him or her. Let your goals be your guide. For people trying to maintain their weight, that may mean a couple of times a month. For others, it may mean less—or more—than that. Some find that richer fare and taste sensations get in the way of the process of changing their palate to simpler, healthier food. People with serious health problems may find they can't afford much, if any, deviation from whole plant foods. Maybe I could be another half inch trimmer in the waist without my occasional others. Maybe not. But it's a system that, for me, has kept mind and body happy. With some experimentation, you'll find what works for you.

PLANT-BASED TRANSFORMATION: JANICE'S JOURNEY

"I want to pull myself out of this hole!" These were the first words Janice spoke to me when we began working together on her transition to eating plant-based. Janice had plenty of reasons to start the journey. "With a family history of diabetes," she explained to me, "I had been told that I was borderline diabetic—and I did not want to end up with the disease. My cholesterol had been up and down, and one of my parents—as well as a grandparent—had type 2 diabetes. I also have a sister who is insulin resistant and on medication. I did not want that to be me. I began reading about various plans and stumbled upon eating plant-based food."

Janice's intentions were to "lose 20 pounds, look and feel better in my clothes, improve my energy levels, sleep better, decrease stress levels, and become solidly footed in plant-based eating for life." She also wanted to "stop being unhappy with myself, like myself more, and be able to be lighthearted." Janice wanted a transformation.

Janice describes two other moments of awakening that inspired her on the plant-based journey. "I was walking one of my dogs one day and for some reason I started thinking about food. I looked down at my dog, and the thought hit me: 'Gee, I wouldn't eat my dog—why do I eat meat?!' Then, I was in the natural foods market and the lady at the checkout stand was noticeably thinner. I remarked on how great she looked. She proceeded to tell me that she had started following a whole food, plant-based diet, which she had read about in a book on sale in their store. I promptly bought that same book, went home, and read through it. The next day I tried some of the recipes and continued trying new recipes from that day forward. I never turned back."

As Janice improved her diet, she enjoyed a growing list of benefits. "I lost 20 pounds, have increased energy, and got back great blood work. I am no longer borderline diabetic. I was amazed at the difference giving up dairy made for my allergies and asthma. And my grocery bill went down."

I asked Janice to name the hardest thing for her in making the shift to plant-based. "I knew this was what I wanted to do, I just didn't know enough about it. So I started reading everything I could. Getting support with a coach made a huge difference. I also really enjoyed reading about how other people did it, and what they ate."

Janice now eats plant foods exclusively, predominantly whole foods with occasional processed treats. She suggests giving up meat, dairy, and oil as soon as you can—and advises referring to a blueprint to help you get started, such as the Seven-Day Plant-Based Journal in this chapter (page 31). Janice said that even though she thinks it's best to "give up everything at the start," her transition to plant-based came in stages. "After about a month of trying some new ideas and recipes, I gave up meats, dairy, oil, and sugar. I still had vegan cookies that were high in oils, though. Those took me two years to give up. I know there are some people who have a hard time giving up certain items—that was mine. Now that I have given those up, I don't even think of them as food, so I don't think about eating them—though I do bake them for my husband. So, bottom line, try to give up everything you can first, though I guess a person's reasons for going on this journey would influence the pace. With my family health history and the problems I was starting to have myself, I knew I needed to make a change quickly."

Janice continues to thrive with the plant-based lifestyle, getting more and more proficient at eating plant-based anywhere—including during family activities and travel to Italy—while enjoying a new lightheartedness and happiness. "I have found that when you are happy," Janice is quick to point out, "it shows in your facial expressions, how you walk, and how you communicate with people in general. I find that I carry myself differently. Along with my weight loss and good health, I have more confidence in me."

CHAPTER 4

The Good News Guide to Hunger Satisfaction

We all know the glorious feeling. Fullness. We crave it, in fact. And once we dig into a meal, we're overwhelmingly compelled to reach it. The question is how to hit those "had enough" hot buttons without giving you beltline remorse the next morning. How do you enjoy being well fed without getting fat? In this chapter we'll elaborate upon how eating whole plant foods from the Plant-Based Plate can help you achieve sustainable weight loss—while still eating until you're satisfied.

Your body has several systems for triggering the fullness mechanism, signaling hunger satisfaction. Three of them are particularly easy to understand. Learning how to leverage them will save you from the untold misery of endless white-knuckle eating restraint. Before divulging the simple details, we'll take a look at the processed continuum, as it plays a major role in the way these systems play out.

You may already have some idea about what constitutes the difference between unprocessed and processed food, unrefined versus refined. Most of us are familiar with wheat bread versus white bread, for example. We understand that one is supposed to be healthier than the other. But what difference does it really make—and what does it all mean for you? How can you be best informed about it, in order to support your quest for superior health and your ideal weight?

THE PROCESSED CONTINUUM

When you hear the phrase "processed foods," what usually comes to mind? For most of us, it conjures up images of cookies, candy, chips, and fast-food restaurant fare. Yet technically, once a food is plucked from a tree or picked from the soil, anything that is done to it before you eat it—chopping, blending, cooking, drying, and grinding, for example—is a form of processing. So if you think about it, most of us actually eat a diet of food that has undergone some form of processing. It's the *degree* of processing that is the important issue.

To clarify the progression—from unprocessed to processed—let's walk wheat through the sequence as an example. The wheat berry is the grain from which wheat flour is made, and it forms the foundation of most breads. Whole grains such as the wheat berry are foods that contain the three components of the seed, or kernel, of the grain: the bran (outer covering), the endosperm (center core of the grain), and the germ (small embryo of the seed). All three parts—synergistically presenting rich nutrition—must be present for a food to be called a whole grain product. Whole grain kernels are harvested and either marketed intact or milled, cracked, or ground—all forms of processing—to produce grain products. The less a whole food is processed, the lower it is on the continuum. The least processed foods we'll call minimally processed. That means they have been marginally altered from their whole, natural state. These are the more desirable—the best match for optimal health and weight. The more a whole food is processed, the higher it is on the continuum, meaning it is more highly processed and potentially more problematic for health and weight.

Here is a progression of whole wheat grain on the processed continuum, in order from least/minimally processed to most refined and processed.

1. **Whole wheat berries: Intact state.**

2. **Cracked whole wheat berries and bulgur: The once intact whole wheat berry has been fractured. The grains are still large; all three parts of the grain are still there, so it's minimally processed.**

3. **Rolled whole wheat flakes:** The whole wheat berry is flattened into thick flakes. All the original parts of the wheat are present.

4. **Stone-ground whole wheat flour and whole wheat flour:** All parts of the wheat berry are present, though the particles are now more finely ground, making it possible to form bread. Stone-ground flour is somewhat coarser—the particles are slightly larger than those in other whole wheat flours—making stone-ground flour slightly less processed.

5. **White flour:** Highly processed and refined. The germ and bran of the original berry are gone, leaving only the endosperm, which has been pulverized to powder for use in baked goods like white bread, commercial pastries, and cookies.

You never suspected that so much could be done with a kernel of wheat. And we didn't even talk about farina, semolina in the form of pasta, or sprouted wheat, which you can find baked into bread in the market. The same continuum can be applied to all grains—oats, barley, corn—starting with the whole grain as found in nature, to fracturing, grinding, and processing to greater degrees until the most refined version spits out at the end.

Why does any of this matter, and why should you focus primarily on inclusion of minimally processed, whole plant foods in your diet? When all parts of the original grain are present, you are enjoying the rich, full nutrition provided by nature. Fiber and other phytonutrients—found only in plants—are maximized in direct proportion to minimal processing. Nothing has been extracted or taken away. The more plant foods are processed and refined, the more nutrition is affected and compromised. The extreme end of the continuum—fractioned, refined fare—can only deliver fractioned nutrition. And we don't get the same benefit from eating food fragments and adding in supplements to make up the difference, either—as much as we might hope chugging bowls of wheat bran and pounding down vitamin pills while noshing on fiber-free pastries will do the trick.

THE WEIGHT LOSS CONNECTION

As you stock your kitchen and get down to the real business of eating, it helps to be mindful of the impact that various degrees of processing might have on your weight. For not only are whole grains more nutritious than highly refined products, but they also serve up a brilliant solution to a perplexing poundage problem. Whole foods help keep you trim when you respect the integrity of them in their whole, or minimally processed, forms. This is partially due to the fact that the rate at which you digest foods is largely determined by their structural integrity. When the intact cell wall of a kernel of whole grain has been too disrupted, your digestive enzymes can get to work digesting and absorbing the now partially unpackaged nutrients with greater ease and speed.[1] Let's take a closer look at why this poses a problem.

As whole foods become increasingly processed and refined, and their complexity is compromised, digestion becomes more *efficient*. Efficiency is usually seen as something positive. Who doesn't want efficiency? Yet when efficiency is used to describe digestion, it means that the ease and rapidity of digestion increase. This means that you are absorbing the energy from the food you eat that much faster. Good, perhaps—if you're trying to gain weight or obtain some quick energy during a marathon. Yet when it comes to weight loss, slowing things down is a distinct benefit. Even if nothing is added or removed—such as when whole grains are ground into whole flours—the properties of the food change. Physically, the grain has been altered from a whole nugget to a course powder, exposing a greater amount of the surface area of the food to your digestive tract, enhancing calorie absorption.

The processing problem is magnified when you run the whole wheat berry all the way through the continuum to the highly refined white flour stage. Now the particles are not only small, but also the food has been fleeced of fiber, resulting in a dustlike powder. This increases the energy concentration of what started out as a quality carbohydrate. Your digestive enzymes now have a field day with rapid digestion, making consumption of a great deal more calories at one sitting a whole lot easier. Compare sitting down to a bowl of old-fashioned oatmeal with a fresh-baked loaf of fluffy white bread. Which is easier to consume—and quickly—potentially beyond your energy intake needs? Refining grains also inspires a higher glucose response. That means a quicker rise in blood sugar accompanied by a rapid drop in same, resulting in a hastened return of your hunger.[2] This can result in increased food consumption and easier weight gain, and can toy with your insulin, triglyceride, and cholesterol levels as well.

The best way to slow down "efficient" digestion is by eating foods close to how they came in nature, rather than refined so much that a grain is merely a shadow of its former whole food self. There is an energy requirement inherent in eating the old-fashioned way, too—chewing whole food—that protects against calorie absorption. The large muscles in your jaw and the work your body undergoes to move fibrous food through your digestive tract demands energy. This workout virtually disappears when chewing and digestion are made easier by mechanically mangling food before it hits your fork.

And let's not forget that when you remove the fiber in food, creating a highly refined product, the calories are not only artificially concentrated in energy but are also now de-concentrated in nutrition. Essentially, gone are pretty much everything but the calories. When carbs get bad press, this is why. The problem is that the media has lumped all starchy carbohydrates together. As you can see, whole foods are an entirely different animal than highly refined carbohydrates, which have been processed beyond recognition.

I ate whole grain bread every day of my 50-pound weight loss. I still enjoy good grainy bread most days. I'm not averse to enjoying a bowl of white rice or pasta on occasion, either. It's what you do 90 percent of the time that matters. Yet armed with the knowledge I have about the impact of the processed continuum, I make sure that the biggest chunk of the grains on my plate are intact or minimally processed.

This same continuum plays out with any other whole food that has been taken through the manufacturing process, which removes fiber, reduces particle size, and otherwise overly refines the food for use in highly processed items such as candy and most cookies, chips, and crackers. These calorie titanics can make a mess of your attempt to satisfy hunger and reach your ideal weight.

THREE RULES OF SATIETY

Eat when you're hungry, stop when you're not. Sounds so simple, doesn't it? Yet to enjoy this kind of eating freedom demands you show respect for the processed continuum in your food choices. This is key to keeping you hunger satisfied and trim. Your body's mechanisms for signaling hunger satisfaction are varied and complex, and no doubt we still have a lot to learn about this intricate interplay of signals between when to eat and when to stop. But we do know that hunger satisfaction is triggered by three important and recognizable elements. I call them weight, stretch, and nutrition.

Weight

We consume just about the same amount of food, in weight, every day.[3] That means if you put all the food you ate today on a platter and weighed it, put all the food you ate yesterday on a platter and weighed it, and so on, each day the platter would weigh about the same. This is why the quality of what you put on that platter matters. A pound of cheese and a pound of potatoes may have the same weight. But which do you think is more likely to cause you to overshoot your energy needs for the day by the time it pushes your weight-of-food hunger satisfaction button? You might logically ask, if you've had enough calories of the higher fat, lower fiber cheese, for example, won't your hunger signals just switch off, telling you that you've had enough? Sorry, it doesn't work that way. Enter rule of satiety number two.

> **BLACK BEANS AND SALAD VS. CHICKEN AND CHEESE**
>
> It can take 3,000–4,000 calories to fill your stomach with chicken and cheese—but only about 400 calories to fill your stomach with a big bowl of salad and black beans. You cannot eat the former foods until you are full, or you're going to have a weight problem.[4]

Stretch

In addition to the weight-of-food phenomenon, you have stretch receptors in your digestive tract that signal to your brain when "just enough" stretch has been hit.[5] When we again compare the cheese and the potatoes, which of these might meet your weight and stretch requirements before you've wildly surpassed your calorie needs? With potatoes—full of fiber—taking up more space at a lower calorie concentration than the cheese, it's potatoes two, cheese zip. Which brings us to the third rule.

Nutrition

Synced with the stretch and weight receptors are nutrient receptors that tell your brain that the nutritional content of your food is adequate.[6] For example, if you eat a pound of vegetable salad, the stretch and weight receptors in your stomach might send the signal that your stomach is full. But the salad might only contain a hundred or so calories, because the space is filled with vegetables that are low in energy density. Though your stomach may be stretched to fire off the stretch receptors, you are not likely to experience an accompanying feeling of satiation—that satisfied "I'm done!" message you get when you've had enough to eat—without nutrition in the form of enough solid energy to back it up. No wonder you're still hungry. That's why trying to subsist on an all-salad regimen won't cut it. You may get the stretch, you may get the weight, but it's too short on calories to provide sufficient energy. Combine that salad with some cooked vegetables and a potato or two, or some rice and beans? Now we're talking. You've just increased the calorie count to a far more satisfactory level—and the nutrient receptors are just as happy as the stretch and weight receptors. See how it works?

WHAT'S FIBER GOT TO DO WITH IT?

In the context of these three rules, you can see why animal products present problems for hunger satisfaction. The same goes for refined food products. Both are waiting for the fiber absolution that never comes. High-fiber plant-based diets are associated with lower body weight.[7] Dietary fiber is a primary player in why the rules of satiety work so well at helping your body stay naturally slim, as fullness is largely a function of sufficient fiber. When foods are fractioned, their composition altered by removing some of their parts, it affects what your body does with them. The implications for weight control are enormous. Fiber is what gives plants their structure—remove it, and you take away a plant's framework. Without fiber, plants would collapse like a house of cards. So does your health.

Interestingly, the part of plants that provides such enormous value to you—fiber—is, at the same time, a part of the plant that your body can't fully digest or hang on to. After you've obtained all the nutrition you can from your food, these nondigestible fibers remain, ready to keep working their post-meal magic. Fiber makes its way largely intact through the rest of your digestive tract before exiting your body. The more fiber you consume via whole plants, the busier the exit door gets. This is a good thing.

There are actually two primary kinds of fiber. Both have properties that are crucial for your health and serve as important agents for easy weight management. Think of fiber as part sponge, part scrub brush. *Insoluble* fiber doesn't dissolve in water, yet hangs on to water in your digestive tract, expanding like a sponge and adding critical bulk to the material moving through your digestive system. Without it, you'd have a major constipation problem. If you've been plant-deficient, this may explain things. The soft mass created by water-soaked fiber is the main reason that plant foods provide you with a feeling of satisfied fullness. This aids easy weight management by taking up digestive tract space and triggering those stretch receptors. *Soluble* fiber, as the name implies, dissolves in water, forming a gel-like substance. It absorbs and holds on to several times its own volume in water, binding with fatty acids and soaking up cholesterol in the small intestine, sweeping it out of your body as waste.[8] Together, this fiber team slows digestion and steadies blood sugar levels, playing a critical role in weight control and reducing the risk of type 2 diabetes.[9] Improving digestion—while functioning as the best natural laxative there is—they speed the excretion of wastes, toxins, and excess hormones from your body.

Our systems were designed for fiber—and lots of it. Most Americans take in a pathetic 15 grams of fiber a day, less than half of the recommended minimum of 38 grams,[10] and barely a fourth of the amount consumed by any card-carrying plant eater. I'm easily in for twice the recommended minimum, a number easy to reach with a bowl of oatmeal, two pieces of fruit, a slice of bread, a tomato, a cup of brown rice, a bowl of salad, a couple of potatoes, a cup of spinach, one and a half cups of green beans, and a bowl of black bean soup. That's almost 70 grams right there. And yes, you do get to eat that much. While there are many fiber supplements available, eating fiber in those isolated forms is not as beneficial as getting it from whole plant foods, which contain thousands of beneficial bioactive compounds that have significant health benefits.[11] To reap the benefits of fiber consumption, get it straight from the plants.

A word of advice. If you have been fiber deficient, hovering around the average of 15 grams a day as most Americans, it may take you a period of adjustment to work your way up to higher fiber content. Too much too soon may cause things to be too loose or windy, back you up, or simply make you very aware of all the new "activity" going on. If so, ease in more slowly. By the time you are ready for the Ten-Day Plant-Based Makeover (page 152), you'll be good to go. (Sorry, couldn't resist.)

Vegetable Oils: Careless Calories?

Marketers have wooed us to value vegetable oil as a healthy diet deity—with a special reverence for olive oil in particular. But truly, what do we have here? An edible substance high in fat—*make that entirely fat*—devoid of the fiber, left behind in the original olive, and a boatload of energy in the form of what could be called careless calories—to the tune of 120-plus for a mere tablespoon.

If questioning the sanctity of olive oil seems like Mediterranean diet sacrilege—we'll talk about that in a minute—you can see why, viewed through the prism of hunger satisfaction and the processed continuum, expelled oils pose a problem for weight management. Taking up very little space in your stomach—yet winning first prize in energy density at 4,000 calories a pound—oil scores low on the satiety scale, and it is shockingly easy to consume. Note that with that 4-tablespoon serving of Newman's Italian you just ladled onto your salad, you are floating in as much fat and as many calories as a serving of Häagen-Dazs.

It's a short step from eating dietary fat to wearing it, and it takes very little energy to go from your fork to your body fat stores. If a researcher were to biopsy the fat deposits of your thigh, abdomen, or pretty much anywhere else that adipose tissue likes to gather, he or she would be able to tell you exactly what kinds of fats you have been eating,[12] and report back to you the dietary origins of your body fat: from chicken, fish, beef, dairy fat, or vegetable oil. Though it is possible for body fat stores to be multiplied via any excessive dietary calorie intake, it is far easier for the body to store dietary fat than dietary carbohydrate as body fat.[13]

I know what you're thinking. "Olive oil is good for you!" and that salad is more filling and stays with you longer when crowned with a dollop of ranch-style dressing. But here's an enlightening nugget that blasts that belief out of the water. High-fat fare, such as vegetable oils, being 100 percent fiber free, do not downshift appetite. By day's end, they just add to your calorie count. In one demonstrative study,[14] fourteen subjects consumed four breakfasts varying in fat and carbohydrate content: one fat-rich low-fiber, one fat-rich high-fiber, one carbohydrate-rich low-fiber, and one carbohydrate-rich high-fiber. Following breakfast, the subjects then left the laboratory and completed appetite ratings at specific times throughout the day. They also recorded all subsequent fluid and food intake. Hands down, the high-fiber carbohydrate-rich breakfast was the winner as the most filling meal, evidenced by less food and energy intake by the study subjects during the morning and at lunch. The high-fat meals were followed by greater food intake through the morning. By day's end, the average total energy intake—calories consumed—was significantly greater following the fat-rich breakfast than after the high-fiber, carbohydrate-rich breakfast.

Not surprisingly, the high-fat breakfasts left eaters cranky and unsatisfied. These meals were not all-you-can-eat. They were matched for calorie content. That means that the high-fat meals took up a lot less plate and stomach space than the low-fat, high-carbohydrate meals to compensate for their higher energy density. The tiny high-fat meal portions added to the dissatisfaction of the subjects in the high-fat meal group. It was as if the high-fat, low-fiber breakfast eaters spent the rest of their day making up for the missing volume and essential carbohydrates that began with the breakfast deficit. Perhaps you know the feeling. As a matter of fact, by the time they finished lunch, all subjects—in all four test conditions—had consumed enough carbohydrates to make up for any breakfast shortfall. The fiber-full, carbohydrate-rich breakfast had already met the need and those subjects sailed through the morning energized and satisfied. These findings are consistent with those from a long list of dietary trials that demonstrate that people eat a constant weight of food—satiety rule number one—regardless of dietary composition.[15,16,17] Can you see the problem here? An increase in the energy density of the diet—as in fat content—results in a passive increased intake of energy. You just eat more to make the weight and stretch match.

Any way you look at it, these results confirm the relatively weak satiating power of fat-rich meals and indicate that high-fiber, carbohydrate-rich meals assist weight control by maintaining fullness. These findings align with results from multiple previous studies, which have shown that a greater amount of energy must be eaten from fat-rich meals than carbohydrate-rich meals before satiation is reached.[18, 19, 20, 21]

What does this mean for you? Dietary fat, with its weak effect on hunger satisfaction, is a risk factor for overconsumption. It means you can't count on the 2 tablespoons of olive oil drizzled on your salad to make you any more hunger satisfied than if you'd done without it. You're still shy of the fiber and other goodies your body is looking for. Basically, it's like giving another 240-calorie load a free pass to your body fat stores, but without the hunger satisfaction. Now you know why portion control doesn't work. Sure, you can try to enjoy being hungry by eating tiny amounts of foods that are so rich in calories that you can't possibly fill yourself, without risking out-eating your energy requirements and stimulating weight gain. But you'll just end up eating more later to make up for it, or fight the urge for hunger satisfaction. The weight of the evidence, considering the rules of satiety and easy storage in your fat cells, makes a strong case for reconsidering oil on your plate. Doing so will have dramatic impact on restoring your naturally healthy weight, not the least of which is the "turn off" effect that low-fat, whole food eating can have on expression of your fat genes.[22]

Mediterranean Mislead

If you began gleefully pouring olive oil all over your plate in response to the popular *New York Times* article "Mediterranean Diet Shown to Ward Off Heart Attack and Stroke!"[23] you were not alone. Extolling the virtues of the Mediterranean diet approach, exhibit A in the article was a study titled "Primary Prevention of Cardiovascular Disease with a Mediterranean Diet."[24] The word "prevention" makes our ears perk up. Add olive oil to the equation and we're off and running for the extra virgin.

On the face of it, the Mediterranean diet approach has a lot going for it: fewer processed foods and high-fat animal products, and increased fruits, vegetables, and whole grains. In this particular study, 7,447 people in Spain who were smokers, were overweight, or had diabetes or other risk factors for heart disease were randomly assigned to follow a) a Mediterranean diet with added olive oil, b) a Mediterranean diet with added nuts, or c) a low-fat diet. Though "no effect on all-cause mortality was apparent," the research showed a correlation between the swap-out of saturated fats for vegetable oils and reduced heart disease. We read "reduced heart disease" and "olive oil" in the article and interpreted that as "eat more oil." Yet even olive oil weighs in at 14 percent saturated fat. All saturated (mostly animal) fat, monounsaturated (olive oil) fat, and polyunsaturated fats are associated with significant increases in new atherosclerotic lesions.[25] Even small amounts of added oils have been shown to have a health-impairing, constrictive effect on blood flow after a meal.[26] Interestingly, olive oil and nut vendors provided the olive oil and nuts for the study. Several of the authors of the study disclosed affiliations in the food and wine industries. Hmm.

It's not a stretch to think that the benefits this study shows are largely due to the reduced intake of animal products and increased consumption of plant foods.[27] The study was not isolated for these elements, so it's hard to say. Certainly noteworthy is the fact that none of these groups demonstrated weight loss—even the group called "low fat." If you're inclined to respond, "See! Low fat doesn't work!" an important clarification is in order. By study's end, in the "low-fat" group, total fat consumption was an insignificant 2 percent lower in dietary fat from calories—at 37 percent—when compared to the other groups. Thirty-seven percent fat does not a "low-fat" diet make. A whole food, plant-based diet, in contrast, delivers roughly 10 percent of its calories from fat in the form of whole plant foods.

RECASTING CALORIES

Here's another piece of good news that may have dawned on you already: Eating whole food, plant-based renders constant calorie counting obsolete. If you've tried an ongoing tally of daily calorie consumption as a way to manage your weight and been frustrated by the results—in addition to the obvious potential mismatch with the rules of satiety—it's because it is not near the exact science you had hoped for. Although awareness of the relative energy concentration inherent in different foods is important, deconstructing everything you eat in a day to a tablespoon of this and a half cup of that is not. Plus, it is wildly imprecise. Not to mention logistically absurd. Yet we are wedded to the clinical "calories in, calories out" paradigm. To be fair, our typical foodstuffs have put us in this position. We are somehow utterly surprised to see our bodies pile on poundage when we do something as natural as eating our fill. It's essential to understand here that it's not your hunger that's the problem; it's how you meet it. In our frustration and attempt to gain some kind of control, we grasp at something we can wrap our head around—numbers. Lured by the apparent certainty of measuring, we relentlessly pursue it in one form or another—whether through counting, portion control, or food exchanges—hooked on the assurance of the calorie count promise. Even the treadmill reassures by counting for us.

Research underscores how eating a plant-based diet promotes weight loss while at the same time liberates you from a dogmatic daily monitoring of calories. One study compared weight lost by subjects randomized into five groups, ranging from a plant-exclusive diet on one end of the spectrum to an omnivorous diet at the other. All groups were instructed to follow low-fat, low-glycemic (indicating the food's effect on a person's blood glucose) guidelines. Participants were free to eat until they were satisfied. At the end of six months, weight loss in the plant-exclusive group—the diet emphasizing vegetables, whole grains, legumes/beans, and fruits—was significantly greater than that in any of the groups that contained meat—pesca-vegetarian (includes fish), semi-vegetarian, and omnivorous—which lost only half as much weight as the plant-exclusive group. Remember, results were obtained without a tedious daily dietary audit, clearly demonstrating a plant-based diet as best match for eating according to hunger and fullness signals while expediting weight loss. The plant-exclusive group also emerged with improved dietary nutrient composition. The weight loss results of this study mirror the health-related outcomes observed in several other large studies.[28] "Completely avoiding all animal products appears to be key for these positive results," notes Gabrielle Turner-McGrievy, lead researcher on the 2014 study published in the journal *Nutrition*. "We've gotten somewhat carb-phobic here in the U.S. when it comes to weight loss," adds McGrievy. "This study might help alleviate the fears of people who enjoy pasta, rice, and other grains but want to lose weight."[29] Further, a 2015 review of fifteen studies, conducted with 755 participants in Europe and the United States, demonstrated that the average person making the switch to a plant-based diet loses about 10 pounds over a period of about forty-four weeks—without calorie counting, or additional exercise.[30]

Yet even "calories in" doesn't tell the whole story about the energy exchange once food is eaten. This is where clinical support for the power of a plant-based diet to maintain naturally healthy weight makes the conversation even juicier. During their studies of populations in rural China,[31] researchers noted that though calorie consumption among the Chinese was significantly *greater* than that of Westerners, the Chinese sported a far lower body mass index. This held true even when adjusted for activity levels. They concluded that diets low in fat and protein, yet high in fiber—the marked observed differences between the U.S. and China populations studied—are associated with lower body weight, *despite higher calorie intake*. In other words, the Chinese were eating more calories and less protein and fat than their U.S. counterparts, yet weighed less. This can be explained by an increased proportion of calories being expended spontaneously in two different ways: 1) calories released as body heat, also known as thermogenesis, and 2) an increase in voluntary physical activity due to an increased urge to move without thinking about it. Over time, these calorie burners add up. After a heavy, high-protein fatty meal—think back to a Thanksgiving feast or two—how inspired were you to suit up for a brisk walk? Compare that to the available energy you might experience following a meal of salad, hearty bean soup, or vegetables and rice. These findings have been consistent with laboratory research in multiple instances[32,33] and in studies with revealing titles such as "Treatment of Obesity with a Low Protein Calorie Unrestricted Diet."[34]

Health and a slender physique can be yours without obsessive micromanagement that sucks the juice out of life in an effort to find the elusive perfect figure. They come delivered on the hunger-satisfying, eat-until-you're-full Plant-Based Plate. With all this good news, why wait another minute to transform your menu—and body? It's time to ready your kitchen so you can get to the fun part: eating!

CHAPTER 5

Getting Your Kitchen and Pantry Ready

"I wish I had been told about the importance of great tools sooner—they made my life so much easier!" Without a moment's hesitation, this was the response of busy mom and business owner Sharon—who brought her husband and three children along to eating plant-exclusive over five years ago—when asked, "What are the top two things you wish you had been told about setting up your kitchen for more plant-based meals?" And that's exactly where we'll go next—to the basic kitchen tools that will make your transition *so much easier*. It's also time to inventory the pantry and fridge, and divest them of inappropriate fare. To help, I've provided a quick lesson on an easy way to wade through food labels.

TOP SEVEN PLANT-BASED KITCHEN COOKING TOOLS

I've found myself in unfamiliar kitchens in foreign countries with nothing more than a subpar knife and a beat-up cooking pot and prepared some simple, glorious, and satisfying repasts—proof positive that you don't need anything fancy to be able to cook plant-based meals. At the same time, there are a couple of common kitchen devices—you may have several already, such as a skillet and a saucepan—that will make mealtime a whole lot quicker and easier. And that means more plant-based meals on your plate and in your body.

Knife and Cutting Board

This point may seem obvious, and you may already have a good knife and board. Yet I start with this pair because they are so fundamental to your enjoyment and ease of food preparation. Above all, a good chopping knife needs to be sharp. My preference is a steel blade with a comfortable handle. I also have a lightweight, thinner-bladed knife that I throw in my checked-in luggage for extended trips—you never know what kind of blade you'll find in that remote Tuscan farmhouse. As for the cutting board, plastic and stone clean up nicely, yet can be tougher on your knife blade than wood. Use what you like.

Food Processor

If speed is one of your objectives, food preparation can be dramatically accelerated with a food processor, which makes it possible for you to rapidly chop, slice, or grate large quantities of vegetables in short order. A food processer is multifunctional and can serve double duty for making bean butters and sandwich fillings, sauces, dips, fruit ice creams, and nut cheese. Find a model that runs quietly and cleans easily. After much research—never stop being a Scout—I purchased a Cuisinart that is a perfect fit.

Pressure Cooker

When it comes to cooking helpers, the starring role would have to go to a pressure cooker. You can do without it, but quite honestly, if you are looking for simple, fast, and delicious—and to make big batches of beans, whole grains, soups, and vegetables, with plenty of leftovers—this item should be in your kitchen arsenal. The pressure cooker has put my old slow cooker out to pasture. But if you have a slow cooker, you can bring it back into business for slow-cooking beans and soups as a good alternative to a pressure cooker.

Find more tips on how to use an electric pressure cooker—including snapshots from my kitchen—at www.theplantbasedjourney.com under Resources.

Rice Cooker

The rice cooker is a low-cost, time- and labor-saving device that, frankly, I'd find it hard to do without. Despite its name, in addition to rice you can cook barley, bulgur, and a lengthy list of delicious grains with it. Simply add the measure of grain and water, push the cook button, and 30 to 40 minutes later—depending on the grain—the cooker will happily chime that your rice is ready. Just to demonstrate its versatility, I've also used my rice cooker to make—surprise—Rice Cooker Baked Apples (page 208).

Blender

A blender can pinch-hit for a food processor, making sauces and bean spreads a breeze, though it won't do the job of grating and chopping that a food grater or processor will. If you have to choose between one or the other, I'd go with a food processor. Once I got mine, my blender was pushed to the back shelf. After several weeks, I pulled it out and it wouldn't start. That was months ago; with the food processor, I don't miss it. I put it in the top five because if you don't have a food processor, the blender is a great gadget for dressings, dips, ice creams, and other quick kitchen creations.

Microwave

The microwave is a time-saver to which you may already be accustomed. Take advantage of your familiarity with it to cook some plant fare: fresh or frozen vegetables, potatoes, sweet potatoes, and yams. Use microwave-safe cookware such as Pyrex, glass, or ceramic dishes marked "heatproof" or "microwave-safe." Covering your food as you cook it in the microwave generates steam heat that is important to the cooking process.

PLANTIFY YOUR PANTRY

At this stage, it is simply a wise choice to remove from your shelves tempting edibles that don't support your new dietary ideal. If your pantry is littered with low-quality snack products—or you have to reach past them to get to real food—when you're in a hurry and push comes to shove, it's easy to guess which might be the default pick. As much as I am a proponent of mental mastery, I'm also a realist. Granted, it would be the highest aspiration for us each to have the equanimity of the Buddha in all food situations. While you're working on that, why push your luck when it's easy to get potential points of risk out of your line of vision? Chips or chocolate—or whatever your personal waterloo—will only hamper your initial progress. Whatever it is that compels you to the cupboard, it's going to call to you, no matter how nicely you ask it not to. If it is a preoccupational hazard, you are probably better off not having it in the house for now.

With a growing understanding of what you will be eating *less* of, it's time to start having fun filling your cupboards and fridge with what you'll be eating *more* of: brown rice and barley, whole grain breads and pastas, black beans and chickpeas, salads and fresh fruits, and vegetables of all kinds. Lots of color everywhere. You want your plate to light up like a Christmas tree. To help you restock, refer to the Shopping List appendix on page 216.

NUTRITION LABELS: THINKING OUTSIDE THE BOX

Problematic ingredients reach beyond the snack food box. The contents lists on everything from innocent-looking soups and cereals to instant meals are getting increasingly lengthy and complex, compounding confusion about what to cook for dinner. How do you decode food labels and run products through the filter of healthy eating?

Your time is at a premium, and it's no wonder the research shows that only a small percentage of shoppers pay attention to nutrition labels.[1] Apparently, even fewer of us know how to interpret them anyway. Plus, who wants a trip to the market to turn into a math project? Food package labels are supposed to enlighten you about the nutrition any given product promises to deliver, so that you can make an informed decision before buying. Yet they're misleading, very subjective, and downright confusing. An in-depth review of the research on the effectiveness of nutrition labels points to one simple conclusion. When it comes to food labels, the best advice I can give you—and the one that will save you the most time and give you the most brilliant results—is to stop trying to figure them out. Instead—and I'll show you how—you can cut through food label clutter and laser in on information that you can use. First, a look at some inherent problems with nutrition labels.

Misleading and Biased

Multiple resources tell you what the different parts of nutrition labels mean. You can find them online at the FDA and several other locations.[2] Yet research underscores the fact that most consumers—the small percentage that actually take the time to read food labels, anyway—have a hard time understanding them. Worldwide, people report being overwhelmed by them.[3] They say they don't have time to process them, they quickly lose interest, and the print's too small anyway. You know the feeling. And if you do have the time and patience to decode them, there's another big problem: A significant shortfall of these labels is that *their numbers are prejudiced*. An example will drive the point home.

The nutrition label pictured below describes a product as having 12 grams of fat per serving. It then states that these 12 grams of fat fulfill "18 percent" of the calories from fat allowed each day "on a 2,000-calorie a day diet." That's the place on the label where you read "percent of daily value." It's also where you'll have to pull out your calculator and start crunching numbers. If 12 grams of fat represent 18 percent of the total daily fat, then five and a half times that 18 percent would equal 100 percent of the daily fat calorie allotment on a 2,000-calorie a day diet, that is. Five and a half times 12 equals 66 grams of fat. Each gram of fat has 9 calories. Nine times 66 equals 584 calories from those 12 grams of fat. Isn't this fun?

I wouldn't take you through all this except for the fact that it makes an important point. Almost there. Five hundred eighty-four calories out of 2,000 calories equals approximately 30 percent. In other words, this entire nutrition label schema is based on the assumption that a diet deriving 30 percent of its calories from fat is ideal. Unless I am aspiring to a 30 percent fat diet, that renders this part of the nutrition label useless. And that's just the fat portion of the program.

To use nutrition labels correctly, for the fats alone, you would need to recalculate everything from the perspective of what a whole food, plant-based

Nutrition Facts

Serving Size 1 cup (228g)
Servings Per Container 2

Amount Per Serving

Calories 250	Calories from Fat 110

	% Daily Value*
Total Fat 12g	**18%**
Saturated Fat 3g	**15%**
Trans Fat 1.5g	
Cholesterol 30mg	**10%**
Sodium 470mg	**20%**
Total Carbohydrate 31g	**10%**
Dietary Fiber 0g	**0%**
Sugars 5g	
Protein 5g	

Vitamin A 4%	•	Vitamin C 2%
Calcium 20%	•	Iron 4%

* Percent Daily Values are based on a 2,000 calorie diet. Your Daily Values may be higher or lower depending on your calorie needs:

	Calories:	2,000	2,500
Total Fat	Less than	65g	80g
Sat Fat	Less than	20g	25g
Cholesterol	Less than	300mg	300mg
Sodium	Less than	2,400mg	2,400mg
Total Carbohydrate		300g	375g
Dietary Fiber		25g	30g

diet naturally delivers—10 to 15 percent of overall dietary calories from fat. Oh, and you'll need to check serving sizes. Which means you have to take into account the exasperating fact that each brand gets to decide—*independently*—what constitutes a serving size. There is no standards regulation. I can make potato chips look pretty low calorie by stating on the label that a "serving size" of potato chips is "one chip." I could go on, though the details only underscore the problems these labels present. My research on decoding food labels also turned up a tutorial or two online. One of them was an eye-glazing nineteen pages long.

Cutting through Label Clutter

Sometimes whole foods do come in packages, but how do you figure out what's actually good for you? Save yourself some time and make it easier by simply jumping to the ingredients that you'll find on the food label—right below the more prominently featured "nutrition facts."

Ingredients in packages are listed on the label in descending order based on weight. The ingredients taking up the most weight in the product are listed first; those with the least are listed last. Without belaboring things, here is a simple four-step guide to help you easily analyze ingredients lists:

1. **Are plant ingredients listed first? Foods with plant ingredients at the top of the list will contain a proportionately greater amount of them relative to other ingredients. If that's what you find, you are off to a good start.**

2. **Is the list short? Having five or fewer ingredients makes the list easy to review and less likely to contain health-harmful hitchhikers.**

3. **Are the ingredients recognizable? Chemical additives, curious flavorings, and artificial anything can easily find their way into packaged foods. If you can't easily decrypt the words on the ingredients list, reconsider.**

4. **Are any of the "crowd these out" items from the Plant-Based Plate (page 30) showing up? Animal products frequently listed are gelatin, along with casein, caseinate, lactalbumin, whey or whey solids, milk solids, and low-fat milk solids—all derived from cow's milk. Albumin is an egg product. "Natural flavoring" on a product can mean flavoring from sources other than those listed—including animal products, unless the label states "vegan" or "animal product free." Avoid added oils. Be wary of lots of added sugar and salt.**

Condiments can be a qualified exception to these rules. Ketchup, mustard, and such represent such a small amount of space on my plate that as long as the labels are free of animal products and oil, and there aren't words I can't pronounce or a list a mile long, I don't obsess about it. Unless you eat ketchup by the cupful, even though a processed product, the amount consumed is usually just as a flavor agent in recipes or as a condiment. Don't sweat the ketchup.

Other than a simple scan of the ingredients, you can gather useful information at the "serving size" and "calories per serving" sections on the label. They tell you that, for example, peanut butter has 200 calories per serving—described as 2 tablespoons. If a serving of peanut butter has meant, for you, a giant scoopful, understanding serving size has important bearing. It informs you that you may be taking in a lot more fat and calories than you thought in that giant scoopful. This is helpful information. When it comes to food labels, there are going to be times when you just want to look away because you don't want to consider that a product is not compatible with your goals—we all do. Just remember, your body doesn't. Look away, that is.

Beware the FOP

The nutrition labels we just examined are on what is known as the BOP—industry-speak for the "back of the package." Now that you know how to navigate that, some fair warning on the front of the package—the FOP. The FOP is where the marketing takes place, and is thus notorious for using misleading language and imagery. In the United States, for example, only pure fruit juice can actually be labeled as "juice." Yet there are several imitation "juice" products that contain no more than 20 percent—or even have a drop of—actual juice. These products are in reality nothing more than sugar solutions pumped up with added flavoring and color. This makes them, in truth, a close relative of cola drinks. Yet they are cleverly named in a way that suggests the real thing—fruit—with words such as "fruit nectar" or "fruit beverage." The illusion is further advanced with innocent-sounding names such as "(Something) Delight."[4]

There's more. Let's say the FOP of the juice box entices you with "made with real berries!" Who doesn't want real berries? Plus, they're high in antioxidants. Toss it in the cart! At this point, being the savvy shopper you are—and knowing that the ingredients label on the back lists items by content amount—you look to the BOP to see whether the FOP claims are what they appear to be. In practice, manufacturers are more likely than not to sell juices that are predominantly apple juice, mixing in other juices in just enough quantity to get you interested. Apple juice is a lot cheaper for the manufacturer to produce than berry juice, yet they know the consumer has been turned on to the benefits of the berry—a fact that they've hooked with the large, colorful image of juicy berries on the FOP. In reality, the juice may only have a smattering of berry. Even as you now know the ingredients are listed by largest amount first, there is no way of knowing what percentage of juice in this product is actually berry juice. Even if the FOP tells you "20 percent real berry juice," what does that mean? Twenty percent of calories? Of weight? Of the wording on the FOP?

One last thing, then I'll rest my case. Internationally there's been hot debate regarding government initiatives to make nutrition label reading easier by implementing a "traffic lights" approach.[5] Green would mean healthy choice, red for questionable—high in sodium and saturated fat, for example—and of course yellow is the caution zone. But who is determining what the green, yellow, and red lights on the packaging mean? And what if the deciding powers rule that green light "healthy" is 30 percent of calories from fat? Houston, we have a problem. And the food industry resists legislated labeling, apparently wanting the freedom to decide how best to disclose the levels of fat, salt, and sugar in their food so that it doesn't damage sales, leaving us at the mercy of the marketing department.[6] We have to take these matters into our own hands and assess food labels with some objectivity. Keep it simple by edging out packages of complex mystery products with real food and the simple packages in which you can have confidence.

Next, it's time to step up to the plate and take eating action. That's what the Rookie stage is all about.

SECTION 3

ROOKIE

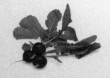

*Stepping Up
to the Plant-Based Plate*

CHAPTER 6

Making the Switch:
Transition Timelines

Now that you have your why, along with shopping list in hand and a well-stocked kitchen, it's time to start actually eating plant-based. But when making the transition to a plant-based lifestyle, what do you think is the best way to go—jump in all at once, or take your time? Overnight overhaul? Or should you make doable changes in small increments, eliminating animal products and processed foods over time? What is the best choice when it comes to pacing? And is one way better than another?

If you answered, "It depends," then you are exactly right. As it turns out, there is no single best pace for the next leg of the journey that is any more right than another. Yet no matter which approach is the best match for you, whether you have the urgency and constitution required for instant makeover or prefer advancing by micro changes—I've seen success with them both—*everyone progresses through each stage of the journey.* These stages are so universal that they are the scaffolding upon which this book is organized. You can't leapfrog over any of these stages and come out ahead. That's why the Scout section is so packed with the details of initial preparedness—your groundwork is not only an asset that has put you at a distinct advantage, but it is also critical to keeping your journey from getting seriously derailed. Now, in the Rookie stage, you'll progress from eating plant-spare to plant-prolific. How far and how fast you advance is your decision. No one's playing food cop here.

SETTING YOUR PACE

To help you establish your own pace, I went to my blog and newsletter readers to find out more about their transitions so that I could share their experiences with you. In my Plant-Based Transition Survey, I asked them, "When making the transition to a plant-based lifestyle, what do you think is the best way to go? Jump in all at once? Or should you make doable changes in smaller increments, such as eliminating animal products and processed foods over time?"

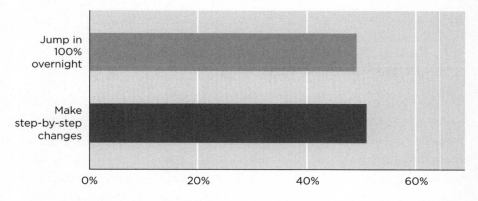

As you can see from the chart, it was a close contest, with the vote for step-by-step leading by a sliver. Yet the responses raised more questions. For example, how long have these responders been successfully eating plant-based? And of those further along the way than others, did one method—jump in or slow and steady—deliver more long-term success than the other?

Almost half of the survey responders had been eating plant-based for at least three years, with some responders already in for ten years, fifteen years, or more. Of the responders who had been eating plant-based for three years or more, slightly more than half reported transitioning gradually over time, similar to the overall survey response.

Yet the plot thickens. Interestingly, of the three-years-or-more group who responded with the advice to "jump in 100 percent and make the transition overnight," a full one-third qualified their answer. In the details, they shared some of the finer points of the stages they went through on their own journey.

They may have jumped in—but in *stages*. This actually translates to a build-upon-small-changes transition, yet rings with the energy of rapid change—just in bites.

> **READER TIP: PREPARE**
>
> Susan Norris from Midlothian, Texas, says: "Jump in 100 percent overnight. Yet I'm going to qualify my response by saying you have to get prepared before you go cold turkey. Get your food lined up, study, and know what you should avoid. I did a twenty-one-day plant-based kick-start and it was rough at first—I didn't know a lot about eating whole food, plant-based and wasn't eating enough. I didn't load up on all the good things I should be eating but concentrated on what to avoid. I'm now more than three years in and the best thing about shifting to this lifestyle is how I feel. Knowing what I eat now is benefiting me and the planet is a real plus, too." Susan is an example of someone who found success by "jumping in"—yet qualified her response with advice to make sure you have taken all the steps to be prepared.

TRANSITION STYLES

The details responders provided regarding the flow of their transitions easily sorted into three different styles: get out of the fire, one at a time, and meal by meal. From these, you can determine the best match for you. Keep in mind that the big qualifier is that you want to choose a transition that will make eating plant-based have *staying power* in your life. I'm not interested in the fastest "success" if it doesn't prove sustainable. That means change that stands up to the critical test of time. Are you overnight or over time?

Get Out of the Fire

Some take what I call the "get out of the fire" approach. Everything on the "avoid" list from the Plant-Based Plate (page 30) is eliminated at once. The upside of this transition style is more immediate benefits and rapid results; the downside is potentially having to deal with any fallout from unexpected circumstances and unpreparedness as it comes up, as is bound to happen with any abrupt change. But that doesn't make this transition technique a deal breaker. It simply underscores the importance of preparation.

For those who turn their lifestyle around overnight in this fashion, frequently it is due to the urgency of illness. Something acute precipitates the change—a heart attack, either personal or of a loved one. A diagnosis of diabetes or other disease can call for immediate action. If your house is going up in flames, you don't look around to see how you can make your house less flammable. You get out of the fire. For others, eagerness and the drive of discovery at the Awakening level inspires them to jump on board fast-track fashion.

READER TIP: CHANGING IN STAGES

"I ended up giving myself a transition period of about two months, in order to learn more about this lifestyle change. I gave up things I shouldn't be eating in stages. Immediately I cut all meat out. Dairy was a bit harder, as I still ate some cheese from time to time. Oil was pretty easy; I only used it sparingly, but eventually did completely away with it. Inside of three months I had dropped nearly 30 pounds. I am all in now and enjoying life! I am interested in what I put in my body, I read labels, and I promote what I am doing for *my* health. If the weight loss and change in my blood work numbers won't convince others, maybe the transformation I am undergoing will."

—*Stephen Toumi*

One at a Time

In the one-at-a-time model, the plant-based journey train clearly pulls out of the depot—your current way of eating. In contrast to all at once, items are phased out in succession on the way to your whole food, plant-predominant destination. For example, some start by excluding meats such as beef and pork, followed by letting go of chicken, then fish. From there, they ditch dairy and eggs—bringing them to animal-product free. Next is quality improvement: switching out highly processed for minimally and unprocessed plant foods. Other people oust undesirables in a different order, first eliminating dairy products and then working their way through the rest of the short list of what to edge out, while increasing consumption of plant foods. In the survey, there were those who immediately eliminated all animal products and then replaced refined foods—a two-terminal approach. There's no singular prescription, and your reasons for going plant-based will no doubt have bearing on your order of operations.

READER TIP: YOU'LL GET THERE!

"I was surprised at how easy meat and dairy were to give up. The hardest part for me still is avoiding the 'junk foods' like French fries and other higher fat items. My biggest challenges were eating enough to stay satisfied and not eating too many processed foods. My advice? Don't be hard on yourself; start with breakfast, then change your lunch. You will get there! You need way less

> fat and protein than you think. Watch *Forks Over Knives*, and read *The China Study*. And build a strong support system—even if it's an online community."
>
> —*Rachael Jacome*

Meal by Meal

An offshoot of the one-at-a-time approach is the one-*meal*-at-a-time system for changing what is now on—or off of—the menu. Meal-by-meal strategists may start by making breakfasts whole food, plant-based, easily fulfilled with, for example, a bowl of oatmeal and fruit, or whole grain toast and fruit, or potatoes and vegetables. Once you get good at that—a week or longer, as needed—you work on lunch, replacing animal products and processed foods with whole plant fare midday. With two out of three meals in a good pattern, it's time to tackle dinner, and all points in between. Of course, you could start with dinner and work your way backward through the day from there. There are a few variations on the theme. There's no right or wrong order. The important thing is getting the mission accomplished.

READER TIP:
A PRAGMATIC APPROACH—AND A 300-POUND WEIGHT LOSS

"I believe that a slow, structured transition toward a plant-based diet is the best approach," says Raymond Cool, down about 300 pounds three years after first setting out on the plant-based journey. "The 'all-or-nothing' approach often results in the 'nothing' half of that proposition. My transition was slow and methodical. By making easier changes at first, it gave me successes to build on—and confidence to make harder changes." Initially quite resistant—Raymond couldn't imagine his life without meat—he was encouraged by the fact that you can eat as many whole grains as you want. "This struck me as something I could do—it was the positive first step I was looking for."

At nearly 500 pounds, rather than making an effort to give up any of his favorite foods, Raymond simply concentrated on eating more whole grains and found them to be delicious, filling, and fun. "I learned how to bake bread, and loved it!" says Raymond. Three months later he found himself several pounds lighter, and couldn't believe how simple and painless it had been to add these healthy foods into his diet. Watching more films about food production and the problems of factory farming edified his journey, and he set out to add even more healthy foods while slowly reducing and finally eliminating meat, dairy, and processed foods—with remarkable results.

Note that each of these strategies demands specific decisions about what there is an increasing quantity of and what's now off the plate. The clarity of your intentions for "in" and "out" is important—even if you progress in stages. Fuzzy, gray areas of action deliver fuzzy, gray results. "Meatless Monday" and the occasional veggie meal, while providing a good point of entry, are not going to deliver the benefits to your health, energy levels, and weight that a plant-predominant menu will. You'll simply never get the chance to enjoy fully the positive outcomes unless you eat a lot more whole plant foods and a lot less of everything else. The more clearly you make the shift, the more results you get. And speaking of results, survey responders overwhelmingly reported that, much to their surprise, they actually now enjoy far more delicious tastes and eating experiences than ever before, now that their eyes and palates have been opened to the new world that eating plant-based delivers.

CIRCLING THE WAGONS: GETTING SUPPORT

Another important way to uplift your journey is to connect with others doing the same thing. Online communities, social media, the buddy system, group classes, private coaching, meetup groups, conferences, and immersion weekends can all be very valuable and important to your success by establishing a support system. Here are a couple of programs that might be a perfect match for you.

Physician's Committee 21-Day Kickstart

The Physicians Committee offers a free twenty-one day online program to get you started on a healthy plant-based diet. Robust resources come with this program: instructional videos, menu plans, recipes, support literature, and an online discussion community where all of your questions are answered by a registered dietitian and Kickstart coaches. A perfect companion to this book, the Kickstart is currently offered each month, starting on the first day of the month, and is also offered in a growing list of languages: English, Spanish, Chinese, Japanese, and Indian.

Find it online: www.21DayKickstart.org

Complete Health Improvement Project

The Complete Health Improvement Project (CHIP) is an affordable, intensive educational lifestyle intervention program offered in community, hospital, and corporate settings. The brainchild of Dr. Hans Diehl, CHIP has attained a worldwide reach of more than 70,000 people since it began twenty-five years ago. A strong feature of the CHIP program is the community-based option. This means you don't have to go anywhere special for a chunk of time or spring for an expensive hotel for a weekend. Classes take place over a few weeks and have the added advantage of helping you practice the skills of plant-based living in your own home with support from instructors, class meetings, and instructional materials. You can check on the CHIP website to see if there is a CHIP program in your area.

Find it online: www.chiphealth.com

Other Resources

There are multiple resources for ongoing education and support for the healthy plant-based lifestyle at www.theplantbasedjourney.com.

• • •

From the survey responders, regardless of transition style, a fundamental theme repeated itself over and over again in their suggestions for success. That is *the importance of preparing for the journey*. Even if you take a jump-in-with-all-fours approach, just like a road trip, you'll need to pack the car and gas up for the journey. That means being fully prepared with what you need so that you don't run out of fuel—food-wise or tactical—before you even get out of Dodge. This underscores the need to pay attention to the initial, essential details of preparation as Scout. Whether "get out of the fire," one-at-a-time, or meal-by-meal sounds like the best match for you, you'll find swap-outs, meal templates, and other success strategies in the next chapters to make your transition even smoother.

PLANT-BASED TRANSFORMATION: JIM'S JOURNEY

Jim's journey is a perfect example of how the urgency of a life-threatening situation can inspire which transition style you choose. After suffering two heart attacks—in the course of a few hours—Jim was ready to grasp the "get out of the fire" option.

Athletic and active for years, Jim let nothing get in the way of outdoor living, including biking, hiking, and otherwise adventuring, on his own, with his wife of forty years, or with his grandson. Jim also loved his food, regularly enjoying steak, meat-based meals, eggs, and all the other hallmarks of a diet heavy in animal products and processed foods. Two years ago, experiencing the clear signs of a serious cardiac event, the then sixty-seven-year-old Jim hastened to his doctor, who confirmed that he had suffered two heart attacks in rapid succession. Rushed by ambulance to the hospital, Jim was scheduled for immediate surgical placement of two stents.

While being prepared for surgery, Jim says, "I asked the doctor—the pre-op IV already in my arm—if there was any possible route I could take to avoid the surgery. His response? 'Not that I know of. We do have a library here at the hospital. You can go up and do some research if you like.'" Jim was rolled into surgery two hours later. Within ten minutes of the completion of surgery, he went into ventricular fibrillation. As a matter of fact, Jim says, "I actually died in the recovery room and came back—the flat line on the monitors was noticed by an observant candy striper." Two days later, Jim, who had always had an aversion to hospitals—and who had found no reason to feel any differently as a result of this experience (he had a terrible reaction to the stents in the form of a hive outbreak, a not uncommon reaction that apparently his doctor hadn't even heard of, increasing his embitterment to the medical establishment)—signed himself out of the hospital and went home. This was strictly against the advice of his attending physician, who warned him, "If you leave right now, you might only have a matter of days to live."

Once home, unsettled by the lack of preventive direction from the medical community, Jim decided to launch an investigation on his own. Googling "reverse heart disease" immediately brought up the book *Prevent and Reverse Heart Disease* by Caldwell B. Esselstyn, MD, which documents one case after another of reversing heart disease with a low-fat, whole food, plant-based diet. According to Esselstyn, as heart disease is a food-borne illness, it's what is flowing through your bloodstream, sourced by what you eat, that counts, even more than the numbers that show up on your lipid profile.[1] Apparently, your food diary trumps your lab work. The photographs of cleared arterial pathways in Esselstyn's book made an impression on Jim, and he immediately embarked on the eating plan. From the start—underpinned by the urgency of his situation—he decided that if he was going to do it, he was going to follow the Esselstyn prescriptive[2] 100 percent. That meant eating all low-fat, whole plant foods—whole grains, legumes, lentils, other vegetables, and fruit.

Soon after Jim's dietary changes, his cholesterol plummeted and his weight dropped from 181 to a lean 135 pounds on his 5-foot-8 frame. His angina a thing of the past, he enthusiastically exclaims that he has never felt better and enjoys his athletic lifestyle more than ever. Understandably, he's become a strong advocate for preventive medicine: "As we all know, though there's no money in it, we need *so* much more in prevention."

Jim now eats and enjoys a variety of plant-based meals, such as polenta and pinto beans with hot sauce and veggies, spinach salad and mixed greens with lunch and dinner, and usually beans and rice for lunch with some kind of vegetable. Jim says, "It was two to three months before I stopped craving fat."

When asked what has been the hardest thing about changing his food plan, Jim responds, "The fact that I had to go it alone." Previously, Jim only shared the cooking duties when it came to barbecue. But Jim's wife did not join him in his dietary change. To this day, there are two lunches and two dinners prepared in their household: the one Jim's wife prepares for herself, still including animal products, and the one Jim prepares for himself. This means his previously enjoyed fare is a constant presence at meals, creating a big challenge for Jim. In addition, Jim says, "What made it initially even more challenging is I had no experience with cooking. It took me some time and experimentation to get the flavors just right. But I'm tough—people are tough—and we do what we want to do. Not even one time have I had a spoonful of meat, eggs, or the other products I know were so damaging to my health."

Jim's wife has experienced some health benefits by association with Jim's cooking. By eating more fruits and vegetables and lighter fare overall, she has dropped 40 pounds in the past year. Still, they share a virtually divided kitchen. I asked Jim his advice on how to stay committed in the face of the challenges of a spouse not coming along on the plant-based journey. "Read the books. Dr. Esselstyn's book gives you actual scientific proof from a cardiac specialist and surgeon," Jim responded. "Stick to your choice by staying connected to the science."

CHAPTER 7
Plant Yourself!

As Rookie, with your transition timeline as your framework, you'll now be moving the yardstick to the next measure of proficiency. You'll make the leap from *learning* to *living* plant-based—and that means simple yet remarkable meals, vibrant well-being, and a slimmer body. No matter which transition style you choose, *simply incorporating more whole plant foods into your diet* is an important action step. You'll start by recognizing and eating more of the plant-based meals you already know and love. Then I'll show you multiple simple strategies for building the presence of plant foods on your plate. This way, you are increasing positive plant-based eating experiences, sorting through new likes and dislikes, tweaking food prep, familiarizing yourself with the plant-based lifestyle landscape, and generally getting the hang of things. This will make the elimination rounds easy.

START WHERE YOU ARE

Transitioning to plant-based eating begins with an awareness of where you are *now*—the point from which you pragmatically move forward. What is on your plate *today*? You'll be happy to discover that there is probably a list of foods you already know and like that are perfectly at home on the Plant-Based Plate. Do you like baked potatoes? Stir-fried vegetables and rice? Most people have had veggie burgers, and dig into them with gusto. What about spaghetti with marinara sauce? Bean burritos and peanut butter sandwiches? These are examples of meals that don't contain animal products (but confirm with a simple check of product labels). You can enjoy them as they are, favorites to bring along with you on the journey. In addition, there are probably several meals you relish that, with just a tweak or two, would be at home on your new Plant-Based Plate.

HOW TO PLANTIFY FAMILIAR FARE

One of the fastest methods for upping your plant foods count is to "plantify" foods that are already favorites. This rapidly expands your list of plant-based meals by taking familiar foods and adding to or swapping out some of the ingredients, shifting their content to more plants in place of animal products or processed foods, and adapting the foods you already like into healthier plant-boosted versions. From these meals, you can develop a roster of familiar, if slightly modified, favorites. This simple four-step activity—*become aware, set your intention, identify,* and *practice*—will show you how. These four steps are fundamental to the change process and elaborated upon in chapter 13, "Mastering Strength of Mind."

> **READER TIP: ENJOY THE FOODS YOU'VE ALWAYS LOVED**
>
> Martha, over a dozen years into whole food, plant-based eating, wisely says, "It's not necessary to make complicated recipes. Keep it simple and enjoy the plant foods you have always loved, which can be more satisfying to eat and time-saving than trying to learn something new and 'strange.' You can always add more pizzazz to recipes later."

Become Aware

For the next three days, make a note of everything you eat—breakfast, lunch, dinner, and snacks. There's no need to write down specific amounts, recipes, or otherwise make judgments. Make it as simple as possible. Don't even press yourself to make any changes yet. You are simply in discovery. At the end of the three days, looking back through your record, find every meal or snack that lives up to your new plant-based ideal. Officially recognize with a star everything on your list that is in alignment with plant-based eating. From this activity, you should become aware of at least a couple of meals you already enjoy that are animal product–free and fairly low in fat. You can organize this list in a folder in your kitchen, on your desk, or on your computer labeled something as simple as "plant-based journey meals." Start eating more of these foods that are a plant-based match.

Set Your Intention

Next, look at the meals next to which you were not able to star as "plant-based." Detect which of these you think will be easy to tweak—strategies for how to do that coming up next—so that they are at home on your growing plant-based meals list. Select a specific meal from your list with which you intend to make adjustments to meet your plant-based ideal.

Identify

Next, identify the specific micro changes you plan to make so that you know exactly which ingredients to be sure to have at the ready. For example, if one of the meals on your favorites list that you were not able to star as "plant-based" is spaghetti with meat sauce, a micro change of replacing the meat sauce with marinara sauce will move this meal into the plant-based category. Identify a specific day—such as tonight's dinner—to prepare it in plant-based fashion.

Practice

Practice preparing more plant-based meals by following through on the dish you decided upon in the previous step. Then, choose another, then another. This is how to build confidence, your file of basic favorites, and a solid go-to list. You simply "plantify" in pragmatic fashion. Soon you will have a solid starting lineup for meals that are going to be a good food fit for you, because they build on the familiar.

READER TIP: THE CONVERT-A-MEAL METHOD

Sandy P., a thirty-one-year-old team sports player from Sydney, Australia— almost seven years plant-based and now a plant-based food blogger—advises: "I think it needs to be emphasized that it's okay to eat simple meals. People can feel overwhelmed and are worried about 'proper nutrition' when they start a plant-based way of eating, yet a simple bowl of rice, veggies, and legumes is great—and not at all hard, either! Think what you used to eat and how can you change that: chicken stir-fry now becomes tofu stir-fry, lasagna with meat sauce now becomes veggie lasagna, Bolognese now becomes lentil Bolognese, split pea and ham soup now becomes split pea and potato soup. I have found this convert-a-meal method has worked great for helping my neighbors and many others, too."

Here are some more examples of how to plantify familiar favorites:

- Taco night is still taco night—simply swap out the meat for refried beans. There's no need to actually fry the beans in oil. Simply mash them up, or slather tortilla shells with Black Bean Chipotle Spread (page 104). Pile on your favorites: tomatoes, lettuce, salsa, onions, avocado, olives, and corn or rice.

- Sandwiches are still sandwiches! Use whole grain bread or pita bread, fill with Hummus (page 103) or other bean spreads, pack with leftover Plant Burgers (page 107), or simply stack with sliced tomatoes and onions, greens, avocado, and some grated carrot.

- Burger night is veggie burger night! Plant Burgers (page 107) have never failed to please. How about grilled portobello mushrooms? Sandwich them in a whole grain bun with all of your favorite burger fixings.

- Burritos aren't just about meat or beans. Potato burritos have become a personal family favorite and make a perfect quick dinner (or breakfast or lunch) using leftover cooked potatoes. Simply steam-fry chopped sweet onions using the Savory Vegetables method (page 99), add cubes of cooked potatoes, and season with your favorite enchilada sauce. Warm tortilla shells or whole wheat chapatis (you can pop them into the microwave in groups for a couple of minutes), spoon in the potato mixture, roll up, and serve with a salad. Or go Indian and season with curry powder and a dab of Cashew Cream (see note on page 196).

Once you get started with swap-outs and thinking outside the standard ingredients box, you'll find that these creative solutions will start to come to you easily. Keep adding to your list and watch a new collection of favorites rapidly emerge.

WONDERFUL WORLD OF NEW TASTES

As you broaden your horizons to the greater world of plant-based foods, you're going to be enjoying a voyage into new taste territory. Some of these flavors you'll take to right away. Some you probably won't like. That's just normal. You can adjust seasonings, or simply give your taste buds an opportunity to make friends with new foods. Working to your advantage is that your taste buds rapidly regenerate on a regular basis. Knowing this can give you confidence as you adventure forward. There's another important element to consider when it comes to taking to the taste transformation on your plate. Your tastes are primarily about *training* and *practice*. Tastes are acquired as opposed to innate, which means they are malleable and can be tweaked to work in your favor. In other words, the foods you eat frequently become your favorites. The more time and distance you put between the foods that you want to move off your plate, the less and less you will miss them—and eventually you will think about them only rarely, if at all.

Speaking from experience—and to demonstrate how you can change your tastes—several years back I had developed the habit of having a piece of dark chocolate after dinner. Nothing wrong with that. Yet, soon, having it at lunch as well seemed like a fine idea. Before long, two pieces sounded good. I knew this practice was probably headed to no good. Though I still eat chocolate, and enjoy it as much as the next person, to change this ritual I swapped out the chocolate for another sweet more compatible with my health and weight goals: Fresh or frozen fruit such as cherries or chunks of mango did the trick. After three or four days, I didn't miss the chocolate. Within a couple of weeks I didn't even think about it. Eventually, the desire for a sweet bite of fruit after each meal faded away as well.

The more heavily processed, seasoned, and high in added fats and sugars your pre-plant-based food plan was, the more plain your new healthy fare might seem in contrast. This is simply due to the taste training you have been experienced while eating your previous food regimen. If you've been eating lots of foods that have been turbo-taste-charged with lots of salt, oil, butter, or sugar, then unadulterated whole food may seem bland. As you start to choose healthy over hyper-enhanced flavor, meal by meal your tastes will respond. The further along the plant-based journey you travel, the more familiar and desirable these new tastes become. And if, by chance, you do stray from your new healthy and now delicious fare, you'll find the food overseasoned and may experience digestive discomfort and a drop in energy from the taxing effect these rich foods have on your body. As unbelievable as it might seem, don't be surprised when the day dawns that you find yourself craving butternut squash or brown rice. Ask any plant-based veteran.

REFLECTIONS OF A FORMER CATTLE RANCHER

"I was raised on a dairy farm—the largest in Montana—and ate meat and potatoes every day. But it wasn't until I changed my diet that I really found out what it was

> to enjoy food. There are more great, tasty foods available once you break the chain of being a meat-and-potato eater than you can imagine. Each day there is no limit to the joy of eating as I now experience it—every day is like a birthday!"
>
> —*Howard Lyman, author of* Mad Cowboy

PLANT PLATE REVOLUTION

The vague directive to "eat more fruits and vegetables" has started to fall on deaf ears. We don't need suggestions; we need specific solutions! The current USDA Dietary Guidelines[1] suggest covering half of your plate with vegetables and fruit, and that the average adult consume a minimum of about seven servings of vegetables and fruits a day along with a similar number of grains. But how often do these show up on *your* plate in comparison?

So here's another strategy to help you move to plant-based meals. Start with the goal of seven-plus servings of vegetables and fruits a day and just as many starchies from the starchy vegetables, whole grains, and beans categories. Make your next plan of action to meet these minimums on most days. And don't worry about doing it all at once on the first day. Bite off as much as you can chew and work your way up. This strategy is extremely effective—even when people don't necessarily have the intention of becoming plant-predominant. Without exception, in my coaching programs, clients who make elevating the status of these foods a priority find that weight loss comes as an easy by-product. By the time you've enjoyed this quantity of whole food goodies over the course of the day, there's little room for anything else. This strategy has such positive results for health and weight that it eventually leads many of my clients to a plant-based lifestyle—as an afterthought.

> **READER TIP: FIVE OR SIX A DAY**
>
> "The most useful advice I got was to eat five or six servings of fruits and vegetables daily. To reach this goal, I eat fruits and vegetables at every meal and as a snack. My preferred snack when at work is a banana—you do not need a container, fork, spoon, or knife!"
>
> —*Jorge, Oregon*

To systematize this, if you are currently eating two helpings of vegetables a day, start by doubling that. If you are eating fruit only every other day, plan and prepare for at least one fruit a day as a start. If your only starchy vegetable is French fries, it doesn't count because French fries get most of their calories from the fat they are fried in, backpedaling any benefit. Change that to a baked potato—with a scoop of salsa on top—and you're in for a starchie *and* a veggie or two. See how it works? Soon you'll not only be meeting the minimums, you'll be surpassing them—crowding the less desirable fare out. Enjoy tracking these counts in a notebook or computer document, simply using checkmarks to congratulate yourself for every whole food, plant-based eating encounter. It's like stars on the chart.

THREE WAYS TO "PLANT" A SANDWICH

Even the Earl of Sandwich, who popularized the idea of something substantial between two pieces of bread, would approve of these variations on the theme. (Whole grain bread always works, though there are other ways to accomplish the sandwich mission.)

1. Stack sliced tomato, thin shavings of red onion, and grated carrots on toasted whole grain bread moistened with mustard or your favorite bean spread.
2. Scoop bean spread, whole grains, or starchy vegetables on large leaves of romaine lettuce, purple cabbage, or steamed collard greens that serve as scoops—roll up, and eat.
3. Pop pieces of Plant Burgers (page 107) into pita bread; add shredded lettuce and carrots or sprouts, some green onion, and a chunk of avocado. You've got a sandwich!

LEGUMES LOVE AFFAIR

Whoever created the old English tale *Jack and the Beanstalk* was on to something when they made magic arrive in the form of beans. This is one affair you *want* to cultivate. Thanks to their synergy of complex carbohydrates, fibers, and plant protein, beans and legumes are practically a prescriptive for promoting satiety and sustainable energy.

FLAVOR INFUSION

My favorite method of bean prep is in the pressure cooker. It's fast, it's sure, and I can infuse them with wonderful, subtle flavors while they cook. A personal favorite is a tablespoon of cumin seeds added to black beans before cooking.

Plant kingdom powerhouses, beans and legumes are practically made for weight management.[2] A bean-rich diet has been associated with a significant reduction in the risk of obesity because beans deliver what is known as the "second meal effect":[3] appetite satisfaction that carries over into subsequent meals, making them the ultimate skinny food.[4] If I can sneak a few beans in at most meals, I can feel the satiety difference. If you've been languishing in bean deficiency, make haste and get the legume light shining brighter on your plate—pronto. Try eating some every day; even one to two cups a day is plenty.

EIGHT EASY WAYS TO LEVERAGE LEGUMES ON YOUR PLATE

1. Pinch-hit Hummus (page 103) for mayo in sandwiches, as a dip for veggies, and thinned with vinegar for a creamy salad dressing.
2. Open a can of pinto beans, rinse, place in a food processor with the "S" blade inserted, add one cup of prepared salsa, and pulse to the desired texture. Heap onto a slice of whole grain toast.
3. Cook Plant Burgers (page 107) in batches and store them in the fridge for a quick addition to salads or sandwiches—or as a convenient meal all by themselves.
4. Scoop Hummus (page 103) on top of any whole grain or potatoes.
5. Open a can of kidney beans or chickpeas, rinse, and add to your salad.
6. Use peanut butter instead of butter on your whole grain toast.
7. Mash black beans—from the can or freezer—spread on a corn or sprouted whole grain tortilla, and top with a little salsa and avocado.
8. Make a batch of Sweet Bean Cream (page 203) and keep it in the fridge to scoop onto your hot cereal or muffins in the morning. Beans at breakfast!

At the same time, if it's been a while since you've been with a bean, it would be wise to work your way up gradually. Beans and other legumes contain enzyme inhibitors that can cause a kerfuffle with your digestive system. Soaking them before cooking helps dismantle the problem, so if you are cooking beans from scratch, soak them overnight before cooking.

Many of us don't have that kind of lead time, however, and there's an easy solution: Simply make sure your beans are completely cooked. You'll know it when the bean easily collapses upon the press of a fork or your tongue, or easily falls apart between a pinch of your fingers. Lentils, split peas, and canned beans tend to be less digestively challenging, canned beans no doubt because they are well cooked—rinse before using to reduce sodium content.

Legumes and beans are so health-promoting and deliver such a massive nutritional return for your investment that it's worthwhile experimenting with ways to work them into your day. Versatile and delicious, this unpretentious plant food hasn't obtained the status it deserves because it is so inexpensive, especially in bulk. You can cook them by the pot and stash servings in the fridge or freezer, saving dollars while shrinking your waistline. The sooner you create a system for daily plantifying via the legume group, the better.

FIVE SUPER-FAST STRATEGIES TO PLANTIFY YOUR PLATE

1. Fold handfuls of chopped spinach or finely shredded Chinese cabbage into brown rice or other freshly cooked whole grains. It will warm and slightly wilt the vegetable, adding a little crunch, color, and all the goods that come with greens.
2. Drop giant handfuls of baby kale into a pot of hot soup, stirring lightly to cook.
3. Drain pasta through a colander and fold in torn fresh spinach or basil leaves.
4. Fold whole kernels of cooked corn and/or chopped red and green peppers into corn bread batter before baking. Extra flavor, a fiesta feel, and more whole plant foods on your plate.
5. Shred carrots and stir into the hummus filling for your sandwich.

By enjoying the foods you have always loved—and adding vegetables you like while leaving out the meat—you start the process of reshaping your tastes. Understanding that tastes are acquired and that we enjoy those flavors with which we are familiar gives you powerful leverage for change as you invite yourself to be accustomed to new tastes. And knowing that you don't need to be perfect in going whole plant foods from day one takes the pressure off.

THE FRONTLOAD EFFECT

When subjects of a clinical trial started a meal with a large salad, not only did their overall consumption of vegetables increase, but also their appetites were moderated as a result. The same fullness effect was achieved by including generous servings of vegetables during the meal. The important thing was to make sure that a robust standard of vegetables was included at some point with the meal.[5] When you load up with fibrous, high-water-content vegetables at the start of—or during—a meal, you can influence how many calories you eat at that meal, an effective strategy for weight management.

To maximize this effect, start with a generous salad or a serving of vegetables rather than waiting until after the main course, so you can enjoy their appetite-satisfying effects. Wait until after the lasagna and bread and it's less likely you'll have room for the slimming side of veggies. That doesn't mean that you need to prepare a big salad and sit down to eat it first at every meal, either. When pressed for time, do what I do—peel a giant carrot, or cut a hearty chunk of cabbage, and munch on it while you prepare the rest of the meal. Any vegetables will do: jicama, sugar snap peas, red bell peppers, and chunks of cauliflower, in any colorful combination. Just think outside the salad bowl and watch your veggie count jump while your waistline shrinks. Vegetable soup has the same effect on calorie consumption at a meal, when served as a first course.[6]

PLANT-BASED TRANSFORMATION: SUSAN'S JOURNEY

Susan's story is a powerful example of the dramatic changes that can result as you patiently commit to changing your tastes, and it clearly illustrates the *become aware, set your intention, identify,* and *practice* strategy. Her tenacity in turning her plant-deficient plate problem around is inspiring and provides a great model for success. A little background on Susan's situation adds to the overall picture.

Susan came to me for help after a year of living perilously when it came to her health. In a very short period of time, Susan had left a job and found herself in the position of needing to provide increasing care for her husband at a level that she found increasingly difficult—and finally impossible—to supply. This on top of the fact that Susan had already became the primary caregiver for her mother. The burden of stress had spiraled Susan's weight upward 15 pounds over the course of a year—with no end in sight. "All the previous year I tried soothing the pressure and stress with vegan junk food," Susan said. "I also began reading books on how to reverse or prevent heart disease and diabetes with a plant-based diet. I was convinced that plant-based was the way to go, and for a while I even convinced myself that I *was* eating plant-based. But now I realize I wasn't." She was desperate to get a grip on the weight climb and restore her previous weight. Susan wisely took action and came to me for help.

Susan understood why a plant-based diet would help her reach her health and weight loss goals. She knew she needed to eat lots of vegetables and fruits along with plenty of starchy vegetables and whole grains. She also had a kitchen well stocked with appropriate food preparation tools and easy, frequent access to markets that were an ideal match for what she needed to put in her cart. So what was the problem? It was time to take a closer look at what was holding her back.

First, I asked Susan if she was aware of any trouble spots during the day. She immediately responded that the hardest time for her was late afternoons, when she wanted to "have a lot of snacks." This was critical information. A review of her food journal—*awareness*—quickly revealed a minefield of mini problems that together spelled out sources of her weight problem and hunger challenges. It showed several sources of hidden fats of which Susan was not aware. Breakfast alone delivered a much higher portion of dietary calories from fats—40 percent—than was compatible with her weight loss goals. And though she wanted to create slimming and satisfying meals, Susan's dislike for fresh fruit, vegetables, and beans were a bit problematic for the plant-based lifestyle aspirant. She recognized that she "did not want to take the time to chew many vegetables," resulting in insufficient vegetable consumption. Clearly, Susan's eating was out of sync with her goals.

To just direct Susan to cut down on the fats and eat more fruits and vegetables would have given her no more information than she already had. She needed specific strategies to shift her meals in a way that would nudge her toward the weight loss she desired, without driving her into deprivation. When it became clear what was getting in the way of her goals, Susan became willing to look at her cemented distaste of fruit, her resistance to taking the time to "chew all those vegetables," and her aversion to beans. She established a clear *intention* to make the changes needed, as she was determined not to let this get in her way of success. Perhaps Susan's progress from awareness of her problem to applying strategies to fix it seems obvious. But that's the thing about habits—they continue to pull us forward, blind to their far-reaching effects and deep impact on our success.

Susan and I worked in step-by-step fashion to deal with these obstacles, *identifying* where specific changes could be implemented and deciding upon specific tactics to address each. Together, these provided just enough change in Susan's regular menu to result in a 10-pound weight loss in our first weeks working together. She completely—yet gradually and in user-friendly fashion—changed her habituated tastes to include more fruits and vegetables, starchies, lower fat options, and less processed food. Without the attention to the small details, Susan would still be stuck with excess poundage and wondering why. Here are some of the important shifts Susan implemented.

First, she started the *practice* of several micro changes that moved her in the direction of her goals. The first was to decrease dietary fat content—starting with breakfast—by cutting back the amount of nuts she had in her oatmeal every morning. Next, she started eating more fruit. Susan's problem with fruits was the texture, and the only fruit she could tolerate was applesauce. She started expanding her fruit repertoire by adding tiny amounts, just a tablespoon at first, of chopped fresh apple to her morning cereal—a micro change in the direction of more fresh fruit. This decision to consciously practice new tastes at breakfast invited Susan to slowly overcome her aversion to the texture of fruit and added to the bulk of her breakfast.

To up her intake of vegetables without necessitating a big salad twice a day—and "all that chewing!"—Susan, a big sandwich fan, was open to the idea of packing as many vegetables into her sandwiches as she could. This was a conscious decision on her part to recalibrate her tastes. Susan's "before" sandwich included two pieces of highly processed bread, several slices of highly processed, plant-derived meat replacement, salt, and pepper. When Susan makes a sandwich now, it is, in her words, "a great big thick thing stuffed with spinach, tomato, bell peppers, sprouts, and hummus."

The practice of plantifying her sandwiches spilled over into other meals as well. Says Susan, "I began doing new things with my food, such as folding grated carrots into my oatmeal. This partially cooked them so that it tasted reminiscent of carrot cake. Salads that previously consisted of mostly cabbage and spinach now include kale, broccoli, tomatoes, sprouts, quinoa, and dressing that is nothing more than my homemade hummus thinned with water."

She also increased her consumption of beans and legumes. "I felt somewhat hampered by my intense dislike of beans. Beans are central to a plant-based diet and I couldn't stand them!" Susan recalls. "I started making my own hummus with garbanzo beans. I tried eggplant hummus with no added oil, only the tahini, and it was delicious. Then I figured out how to make my own. I ate lentils. Didn't like them before. Then Lani suggested sprouting them and adding them to my salads, and they were great!"

"This has resulted in more success than I even imagined," Susan continues. "I wanted to lose the extra 15 pounds, but I also wanted to avoid the health problems I was seeing in the people around me every day. I didn't want to end up with dementia, heart disease, diabetes, or any of the other lifestyle diseases that my husband suffered from. I don't want to spend the last twenty years of my life in misery, taking pills, seeing doctors, and being a proud owner of a handicap parking placard. That actually became more important than losing the extra weight. Not only am I now down a dozen pounds, but I've also learned a lot more about the plant-based lifestyle and know that what I eat nowadays really is low fat and plant-based. Compared to a few months ago, I feel so much better—in absolutely every way."

CHAPTER 8
Creating Systems for Success

Swap-outs—and otherwise plantifying familiar meal favorites, as you have started to do—create *systems* that ultimately translate to transition to a plant-based diet. Setting up systems that support your journey accelerates your progress. Systems establish efficiency and ease for successful change, just as they do in any endeavor—by setting up the ways and means for you to easily take action, over and over again. Systematize food readiness by leveraging meal planners, go-to meals, and recipe templates. In this chapter I'll provide you with all of these and more.

SIMPLICITY AND PREPAREDNESS

Strategies for organizing and consolidating your food prep time keep your new way of eating from becoming overwhelming. Whether your style is "out-of-the-fire," one at a time, or meal-by-meal, simplicity and preparedness are the two principles on which your transition success—and all of the instructions provided at this stage—are based.

On the plant-based transitions survey, I asked readers to share what they wish they had known when starting their journey. Over and over again, the responses delivered this message: *Learn how to keep it simple* and *learn how to prepare*. They are the secrets to easy, efficient meal planning and preparation. Being prepared helps you *keep* it simple.

> **READER TIP: KEEP IT SIMPLE**
>
> "My top tip for someone embarking on the plant-based journey? Make it as simple as possible. You don't have to cook elaborate meals. Have a baked potato or sweet potato, a salad with vinegar for dressing, and fresh fruit for dessert!"
>
> —*Kim M., North Carolina*

MORE SYSTEMS FOR MEAL READINESS

If you find yourself scrambling at the last minute, scratching your head about what's for dinner while you're famished or stressed at the end of a busy day, you're doomed. The best way to show support for yourself is by being prepared beforehand. Readying food in advance, either on the weekend or at some other planned time during the week—chopping veggies, washing potatoes, or cooking a big pot of oats in the slow cooker for easy heating in the morning—can make all the difference between following through and falling away.

University activities planner, grandmother, and gardening enthusiast Nancy M. has preparation nailed. She has developed a system she calls her "every Sunday things." That way she has food ready for her busy week, and just has to grab and go. See if her Sunday ritual would work for you—or let it inspire your own method.

- Clean and chop lettuce.
- Cut up green onions.
- Have mushrooms or grape or cherry tomatoes on hand.
- Rinse canned chickpeas or black beans, and place in a container in the fridge.
- Slice zucchini, cucumbers, or yellow squash.
- Cut up carrots and make a container of homemade hummus for dipping.
- Cook eight or ten potatoes in the pressure cooker.
- Cook a batch of brown rice, separate into serving sizes, and freeze.
- Make individual servings of vegetable shepherd's pie and freeze.
- Make a big batch of sweet potato black bean enchiladas, separate, and freeze.

See the wisdom in Nancy's system? She has a flavorful assortment of foods ready to go. That means during the busy week, Nancy's food prep is basically done. Preparation in advance saves you when you're rushed, which is always going to be far more often than you think. By doing some prep beforehand, making meals takes only a short time, because the most time-consuming work is already done.

• • •

Like Nancy, I can open my fridge just about any day of the week and find everything I need ready to go for fast meal preparation: cooked brown rice; baked potatoes or yams; cooked beans; prewashed bags of baby spinach, romaine lettuce, or both; cabbage; tomatoes; several pounds of carrots; red bell peppers; bunches of kale; broccoli; apples; tofu; frozen corn and peas; and frozen blueberries and mangoes or cherries. From this short list, together with an item or two I might grab from the pantry, I can pull together at least a dozen different meals.

READER TIPS: NINA'S TOP FIVE FOR PEOPLE STARTING OUT

1. Start with one or two new recipes per week. With so many recipes online you don't have to buy every single plant-based cookbook on the market. Just buy one and focus on it for a while!
2. When going out to eat, choose a restaurant that has international cuisine: Chinese, Japanese, Thai, or Italian. There will be more plant-based options on the menu.
3. Prepare food for the week on Sunday and have healthy snacks on hand that are washed and ready to go for when you start to have a craving—or you're plain and simple hungry!
4. Take a cooking class from someone who teaches plant-based cooking, such as the fine folks from Physician's Committee. The instructor does all the cooking, and you get to taste the food and take the recipes home! These classes are affordable and a great way to learn just how easy a plant-based diet can be.
5. Add in more of the good stuff, while minimizing the "bad" stuff! Going plant-based has completely changed my life. I had my blood tested before I started, and a year later my immune system was significantly stronger. As an elementary school teacher, I work in a Petri dish of germs—yet I am rarely sick! I am forever grateful for having made this transition.

—Nina Osberg, Washington

PLANT-BASED MEAL-PLANNING SYSTEMS

Going from zero to all whole food, plant-based menus in one acceleration can seem mind-boggling when you are used to the mind-set of "get your protein here, your carbs there, and your fats somewhere else." Meal planning can present similar challenges if this has been your frame of reference. Seeing your food as a synergistic presentation of whole plant nutrients overrides the macronutrient paradigm, yet can understandably seem destabilizing to the meal-planning process to which you may be accustomed. Although you can't "unlearn" anything, when you start to appreciate the nutritional riches that plant foods deliver, the paralyzing grip of the "square meal" starts to loosen, and the relaxed pleasure of mealtime is restored. As you advance on the plant-based journey, it will become easier to think beyond the isolated nutrient paradigm to the new one: whole food. Here are two meal-planning strategies that will help, starting with the simplest.

"End of the Day Platter" Meal Plan

If I were to take all the food I eat on any given day and heap it onto one big platter, about half of the platter would be stacked with colorful nonstarchy vegetables—some cooked, some raw—and a few pieces of fruit. The other half would be filled with an assortment of robust whole grains, starchy vegetables, beans, and legumes. Sprinkled over the top would be some seeds or nuts. You'd spot a few decorations in the form of condiments, simple dressings, or sauces. That's my meal plan—the "end of the day platter" plan. These meals show up as an assortment of overstuffed sandwiches, simple salad mountains, aromatic rices and legumes, festive veggie wraps, enticing bowls of chili with sweet corn bread, colorful stacks of steamy greens, filling enchiladas, savory soups, and stir-fries. I'm always aspiring to more leafy greens and variety. That's as complex as it gets. I don't measure it, obsess about the balance, or otherwise micromanage my plate. And you needn't, either. Keep whole plant foods, minimally processed, as your guide. Eat abundantly according to appetite from the five food groups, being generally mindful of the composition of the "end of the day platter" snapshot that's the best match for you. Eat enough to keep up with your energy needs and for full hunger satisfaction.

> **READER TIP: "GOOD ENOUGH"**
>
> "Plant-based eating does not have to be complicated to be interesting. Eating a plant-based diet is a journey. That means there are twists and turns and trying to be 'perfect' is counterproductive. Be 'good enough' in your choices and you'll find yourself getting closer—and happier."
>
> —*Martha, Colorado*

Easy Plant-Based Meal Planner

Although the sage advice from the plant-based physicians and dietitians to "just eat from a variety of whole plant foods over the course of the day, and you'll have everything you need" may be true, it might feel a little bit too freewheeling for you—as if your ship's been sent to sea without a rudder. After all, many of us grew up with one variation or another of Mom's "main course, vegetable, and a fruit" meal-planning model. No wonder "just eat from a variety of" might seem like too much of a jump off a cliff. It's understandable that you might need a little more structure as you get started. The Easy Meal Planner merges conventional meal planning with the plant-based perspective, bridging the gap.

My mom planned meals that way, too—main course, vegetable, and fruit. So I understand the urge to create some kind of connection between what you may already know about meals and the shifts you want to make. Actually, your instincts are good, as that is how we learn—by linking new information with patterns from the past. Instead of just throwing everything out the window—and trying to get comfortable with it—why not take the ideas you may already have about meal planning and overlay "plant-based" for a comfortable fit? You may have all you need with my model of "end of the day platter" imagery. Yet if you need something more concrete, the Easy Meal Planner might give you more confidence. And if the "main course, vegetable, fruit" model is not part of your experience, it provides you with a structure.

> **READER TIP: MEAL PLANNING**
>
> Shana S. says, "I remember when I started cooking plant-based—sitting and staring at a blank page because I didn't know how to menu plan or grocery shop without starting with a main dish based around meat. Meat alternatives helped me get started on my journey."

Here's how the Easy Meal Planner works. To easily build a dinner menu by adapting the main course-vegetable-fruit model, instead of the old meat loaf and mashed potatoes, burger and fries, or chicken with rice, a plant-based main course might be black bean soup with a chunk of good grainy bread, lentil curry over rice, a bean burrito, a Plant Burger (page 107) with the works, or a baked potato smothered in red lentil sauce. For the vegetable? A large salad, heap of fragrant steamed vegetables, or both; stir-fried vegetables to go with the brown rice and black beans; some vegetables cooked into your soup; or simply carrot and celery sticks with bean dip. Fresh fruit—chopped, sliced, or whole—serves as the perfect finish. For example, rice and beans, a salad, and sliced orange comprise a complete dinner Easy Meal Planner style.

What about lunch? A Hummus (page 103) sandwich with sliced tomato, starring the chickpeas in the hummus and the whole grains in your bread or wrap for your main dish. Cabbage slaw comes along for the ride as a vegetable, and a crisp apple now or later. This is as complex as your meal planning ever need get. It's an excellent way to satisfy the need for a simple structure for eating, while keeping your meal-planning mind happy. What started out as "main course-vegetable-fruit" is now second nature, and you'll be able to pull a simple meal together with one hand behind your back. If you take a look back at the Plant-Based Journal on page 30, you'll see this kind of structure all over the place. Pretty much every lunch and dinner reflects this rhythm.

The Easy Meal Planner allows you to see your previous ideas about meal plans in a plant-based context. You take care of your nutrition needs for the day by remembering legumes, whole grains and starchy vegetables, nonstarchy vegetables, and fruit at lunch and/or dinner—or simply at some point in between. While staying mindful of eating plenty of everything, you'll soon learn that the sky won't fall if a bean or grain doesn't make it to every single meal. It's what you are eating over the course of a few days that matters. Just think whole plant food, and keep the image of plenty of vegetables and fruits and sufficient starchies to balance out your end-of-the-day platter in mind. With the meal-planning guide as easy reference, you have a specific starting point directly connected to what you want to achieve—eating plant-based.

Here are some examples of simple dinners implementing the Easy Meal Planner. Beneath the menu, in the left column, is the meal plan component, the center column is the specific whole plant food item that fulfills that role in the plan, and the column on the right briefly describes the preparation method.

Easy Meal Planner Sample #1

Menu: Red lentil curry with brown jasmine rice; savory summer squash and mushrooms; apple

Meal Component	Whole Plant Food	Preparation Method
Main course	Red lentil curry served over brown jasmine rice	Cook the red lentils by simmering on the stove, in the pressure cooker, or in the slow cooker, adding your favorite curry seasoning during cooking. Cook the brown rice in a rice cooker.
Vegetable	Summer squash, sweet onions, and mushrooms	Cook according to the Savory Vegetables Template (page 99).
Fruit	Apple	Either eat whole, slice, or serve as Rice Cooker Baked Apples (page 208), or save it for later.

In order to make a week of similar dinners using the Easy Meal Planner Sample #1, you could simply make sure that you have on hand:

1. **Starchy vegetables and whole grains for five to seven meals. Stock up with a pot of potatoes and a large batch of brown rice or other whole grain that you can store in the refrigerator and eat for a couple of days. Replenish with another batch—or mix in barley, bulgur, or any other whole grain and starchy vegetable such as potatoes—as needed. The trick is having this already cooked and ready as backup in the fridge, or poised to go at the push of the rice cooker, oven, or pressure cooker button.**

2. **Beans and legumes that you can serve over the starchy vegetable or whole grain, on a salad, or cooked into a soup or chili. Have several cans of beans on hand, and as you get the hang of it, you'll be able to cook larger batches of beans to keep in the fridge or stash in your freezer, where they will keep much longer. You simply have to get them out to thaw in time.**

3. **A variety of vegetables to go with the starchy vegetables or whole grains, such as cauliflower, zucchini, broccoli, bok choy, Swiss chard, summer squash, spinach, onions, and kale. Keep your favorite vegetable backups in the freezer. The Savory Vegetables Template (page 99) is a system that keeps cooking ultra-simple. You could also elect to cook the vegetables in a pressure cooker (3 to 6 minutes), steamer, or oven.**

As an alternative, you could swap out the cooked vegetables in Planner #1 for salad or simply add a salad to the meal. Keep leafy greens such as baby spinach, romaine, arugula, or cabbage on hand for daily salads. Prepare from either whole heads of lettuce or cabbage, or use bags of prepared, washed greens. You can keep your salad simple greens or decorate with other vegetables or beans. Start with your favorites and gradually branch out from there as you invite yourself to add more colors and expand your taste repertoire.

You can see how easy it is going to be to meet your seven vegetable servings goal. With this meal planner, featuring two or more cups of savory vegetables, you are easily in for four or five servings of vegetables at dinner alone.

Easy Meal Planner Sample #2

Menu: Plant Burger (page 107) on whole grain bun; romaine lettuce salad; fresh fruit salad

Meal Component	Whole Plant Food	Preparation Method
Main course	Plant Burger: All American served on whole grain bun	Cook burger according to recipe on page 107, or reheat already cooked burger in a pan; toast or grill the bun.
Vegetable	Salad of romaine lettuce Extra veggies: Tomatoes, onions, leafy lettuce	Tear romaine lettuce into bite-size pieces. Top with Sweet and Sour Dressing (page 202). Slice the extra veggies and top your burger with them.
Fruit	Apple and banana fruit salad	Chop the apple and banana, and serve in a bowl or save for later.

Easy Meal Plan Sample #3

Menu: Simple Vegetable Soup (page 114); spinach salad with leftover Golden Turmeric Rice (page 195); sliced orange

Meal Component	Whole Plant Food	Preparation Method
Main course	Simple Vegetable Soup	Prepare the soup according to the recipe on page 114.
Vegetable	Spinach salad; vegetables in the soup	Tear spinach into bite-size pieces and pile in bowl or on a plate. This provides a perfect base for a scoop of Golden Turmeric Rice. Serve with sweet balsamic vinegar.
Fruit	Fresh orange	Peel, slice, and serve on a plate or save for later.

Easy Meal Plan Sample #4

Menu: Hummus sandwich with extra vegetables on the side; cherries

Meal Component	Whole Plant Food	Preparation Method
Main course	Hummus on whole grain or pita bread	Spread Hummus (page 103) on bread or stuff into pita.
Vegetable	Cucumbers, shredded lettuce, and tomatoes	Slice the cucumbers and tomatoes, and shred the lettuce if desired. Add to the sandwich or pita.
Fruit	Cherries	Serve on the side or save for later.

MOCK MEATS

What about those commercial foods that mimic animal products in the form of luncheon meats, burger-like crumbles, or vegetarian hot dogs? These foods can be useful for company and fun on special occasions. They do present value as "transition" foods because they can be reminiscent of meat in texture and flavor. At the same time, these foods are usually highly processed, lacking in fiber, and often high in sodium and fat. Once they've fulfilled a transitional purpose, it's better to eat them only occasionally, keeping your eyes on the prize: whole plant foods.

You can ease into the plant-eater lifestyle by preparing simple meals like these without putting pressure on yourself to cook fancy recipes. To be honest, my idea of the perfect recipe is one with five ingredients or fewer. I like to get meals ready with as little fuss as possible so that I can get on to the fun part—eating. And unless you want to, you don't have to become a gourmet cook to eat well. The expectations are too great and you just risk burning yourself out and collapsing under the pressure. Tiptoe into new recipes as you have the time or inclination. Trying out a new recipe on a Saturday can be a good way to increase your repertoire and build confidence in the kitchen. To help, I have provided several recipes in chapter 14, along with a list of cookbooks in the Resources section of www.theplantbasedjourney.com. No matter how you cook, you will discover new tastes and ingredients to your liking. Over time, these will become your new staples.

Recipe *templates*—several of which I've provided for you here—give you another simple system of food prep, helping you shift out of the mind-set of needing to make over-the-top recipes for each meal.

READER TIP: HANDY RECIPE LOCATOR

"Make a recipe locater index on your computer! Learning to cook new things means finding all sorts of new recipes from multiple sources—magazines, cookbooks, online websites, blogs, etc.

"If you are like me, you will remember cooking that scrumptious eggless lemon cake, but when it's time to make it again, you may not be able to locate the recipe. When you make a dish you like, record the name and where you got it in some sort of file. This can be Pinterest, or just on a notebook somewhere. I keep track of recipes that I have tested and think would work well for company in this same folder."

—Janet Bacon, Colorado
(five years plant-based—now studying to become a registered dietitian)

"GO-TO" MEALS

With the help of the Easy Meal Planner and insights about how to be prepared with what you need for eating delicious and satisfying meals day in and day out, you'll soon discover that you have assembled a list of "go-to" meals. Most of us cycle meal favorites. This means we usually rotate among two or three breakfast options, three or four lunches, and five or six dinners. Simply select your favorites of these meals—in a plant-based context—build your repertoire, and there you have it: your go-to list of reliable eats. Then, as you start to gain confidence with what a plant-centric plate looks like, you can try new combinations and recipes.

FIVE OF MY TOP GO-TO MEALS
1. Golden Turmeric Rice (page 195) served with steamed broccoli.
2. Red or gold potatoes dressed with salsa and baby spinach salad topped with red beans.
3. Brown jasmine rice with lentil curry and Savory Vegetables (page 99).
4. Avocado/onion/tomato sandwich with Hummus (page 103) on whole grain bread.
5. Plant Burgers (page 107) and romaine lettuce tossed with Sweet and Sour Dressing (page 202).

PLANT-BASED RECIPE TEMPLATES

Recipe templates make plant-based prep easy. Here are several that I implement over and over again. All you need to do is switch out the main players for an endless variety of options. The template method meets the need expressed by many people who say that when they got started with plant-based eating, they wished they had not felt it was necessary to make fancy meals or complex recipes to do it "right." They wanted something simple. Plus, it's the way I cook most of the time.

READER TIP: SOME OF THE BEST MEALS

Thirty-six-year-old high school library secretary Lisa D. has been a vegetarian for nine years and plant-exclusive for almost five. "Cookbooks are good for inspiration, but can sometimes be discouraging with long lists of ingredients, some of which can be unusual or hard to find," says Lisa. "There's nothing wrong with a simple grain-bean-vegetable meal flavored with herbs, spices, vinegars, or other seasonings. Also, cooking without recipes can lead to some of the best meals!"

WHOLE GRAIN BREAKFAST TEMPLATE: OATMEAL AND APPLES

This delicious and edifying breakfast is such a plant-based basic, I would be remiss not to outline here how simple it is to make. You may think that everyone knows how to prepare a big bowl of oatmeal, but that's not necessarily the case.

- 3–4   cups water, depending on the consistency you prefer
- 1½   cups uncooked old-fashioned rolled or steel-cut oats
- 1   large crisp apple, chopped (or 1–1½ cups of any fruit you like)
  Splash of plant milk
  Sprinkle of cinnamon or other seasoning to taste

1. Bring the water to a boil in a medium saucepan. Add the oats, reduce the heat, and cook for 10 minutes (for rolled oats) to 20 minutes (for steel-cut), stirring occasionally. Cover, remove from the heat, and let stand for a few minutes before serving.

2. Pour the cooked oats into a serving dish and top with the apple, plant milk, and cinnamon. Serve.

YIELD: 2 generous servings

NOTES

SERVING OPTIONS: You can also decorate with a sprinkling of raisins, walnuts, or a teaspoon of brown sugar or maple syrup.

MICROWAVE COOKING METHOD: Steel-cut oats cook more slowly than old-fashioned oats. You can also cook both rather quickly in the microwave. For microwave cooking:

1. Place the oats and water in a large glass or Pyrex bowl.
2. Cook on high for 4 minutes. If cooking the rolled oats, they will be ready. For the steel-cut oats, after the initial 4 minutes, let the bowl sit for 10 minutes, then stir and cook again on high for 2 more minutes and let it sit for 5 minutes before serving.

EVENING PREP METHOD FOR A FASTER BREAKFAST: To save time in the morning, oats can be partially cooked the night before either in the microwave or on the stove top, covered, and left to sit overnight on the counter. Finish cooking in the morning.

NO-COOK METHOD: Simply soaking old-fashioned rolled oats for 15 minutes or overnight makes them ready for eating—no cooking required. Scoop the amount of oats you'd like to serve into individual bowls or one large bowl, cover with plant milk or hot water, and you have softened, ready-to-chew sweet oats. Add fruit and the optional splash of plant milk to complete your breakfast.

EASY VARIATION IDEAS: To make whole grain breakfast variations, simply swap out the fruit, grain, and seasonings. Some of my favorite variations on oatmeal using other whole grains are cream of rice and polenta. These are cooked in the same fashion as the oats with one exception: They need a little more water. For these hot cereals made of coarsely ground grains, use roughly one part grain to four parts water. Adjust cooking times and water-to-grain ratios to suit your taste.

BREAKFAST

Some people swear by breakfast, and others say they never touch it. Which practice is best when it comes to health and weight management? Often "no appetite at breakfast" translates to "I ate too much last night." Here's the problem this presents. The day begins, you pass on early eats due to lack of appetite, and before you know it it's 10:00 A.M., you're famished, and good food choices are nowhere in sight—trouble. The solution? Simply plan for a solid, healthy plant-based breakfast whenever the need hits. You can take your whole grains, oatmeal, and fruit in a container with you, all ready to go when you get hungry. Burritos, hummus sandwiches, vegetables and bean spread, cold baked potatoes, and leftovers also make excellent breakfasts.

Perhaps your problem is that you are so rushed in the morning that you've let breakfast become an afterthought. The key to a good breakfast—one that is healthy and robust enough to launch an energetic, appetite-stable day—is forethought. Planning, and even going so far as cooking—a good breakfast the night before, so that it's ready on demand the next morning when you are in a hurry, is the sign of a Champion.

✴ ✴ ✴ ✴ ✴ VARIATIONS ✴ ✴ ✴ ✴ ✴

Whole Grain Breakfast Template Variation: Peachy Quinoa

You can't beat the visual feast of red quinoa decorated with the luscious pinkish orange of peaches or nectarines for this breakfast. Whole grain breakfasts don't have to be hot—and this meal works wonderfully cold. I like to cook the quinoa in advance and chill in the refrigerator overnight.

   3   cups water
   1½ cups red quinoa
   1½ cups sliced peaches
   2   tablespoons chopped walnuts
       Splash of plant milk

1. To cook the quinoa, bring the water and quinoa to a boil in a medium saucepan. Reduce the heat to low, cover, and simmer until tender and most of the liquid has been absorbed, 15 to 20 minutes. Fluff with a fork.

2. Stir in the peaches, walnuts, and plant milk. Serve.

YIELD: 2 servings

QUINOA

Quinoa is gluten-free and more concentrated in protein and calcium than most other grains. Actually, although quinoa functions in meals in a fashion similar to grains, it is actually a seed. Because its particles are smaller, quinoa—both the light yellow and the dark red varieties—cooks conveniently faster than do whole grains. Very versatile—as are most whole grains—quinoa is comfortable at breakfast, lunch, or dinner.

SAVORY VEGETABLES TEMPLATE

With this simple system you will be able to quickly prepare rich savory vegetables without the addition of vegetable oil. The key to cooking vegetables in this fashion is to add the broth a few tablespoons at a time as the vegetables cook, so that you sauté and caramelize rather than boil them, enhancing flavor.

1–1½ cups vegetable broth
   1 sweet onion, diced
   2 cloves garlic, pressed, or 1 teaspoon garlic powder
1–2 tablespoons seasoning of your choice, to taste, in any combination (ex: curry, smoky paprika)
4–5 cups chunked or sliced vegetables of your choice (ex: broccoli and red peppers, cauliflower and corn, zucchini and eggplant, green beans and mushrooms)
   Salt and freshly ground pepper, to taste

1. Splash a couple of tablespoons of the vegetable broth into a 2-quart stainless-steel pan and start to cook over medium heat.

2. Add the onions and garlic and cook, stirring, for a few minutes until they brown around the edges and the onions start to caramelize and turn golden. Stir in the seasonings.

3. Add the rest of the vegetables in order of cooking time needed. (For example, because mushrooms cook much faster than green beans do, if cooking a green bean/mushroom combination, add the green beans first so that they finish cooking at the same time as the mushrooms.)

4. Once all the vegetables have been added, place the lid on the pan and turn down the heat to low. Keep an eye on the process—as the broth cooks down, you may need to add more so that the vegetables don't start to stick to the bottom of the pan. Normally you will need to add more broth a couple of times during the cooking process, 2–3 tablespoons at a time.

5. Serve with salt and pepper over grains, potatoes, pasta, or simply alone.

YIELD: 2 servings

NOTE

This template provides you with the framework for endless meal options, such as summer squash, onions, and mushrooms seasoned with curry and served over brown jasmine rice, or cauliflower and onions served with quinoa and Creamy Corn

Sauce (page 101). Start with your favorite vegetables, whole grains, and sauces for making simple, satisfying meals.

WHAT ABOUT SALT?

Our tastes have become accustomed to the high salt content in packaged products and restaurant meals. While a little bit of salt can be very helpful in increasing your enjoyment of healthy ingredients such as vegetables and whole grains, as you prepare more foods at home, your tastes will adjust and you will find yourself using less salt altogether. Before long, restaurant fare may seem far too salty.

If you do salt your food at home, experiment with adding it after cooking by sprinkling it on the surface of your dishes. This way, the taste is more readily detected and far less is needed. The salt in these recipes is always optional, and you are in control of how much salt you use. Products such as low-sodium miso and tamari are lower in sodium yet richer in flavor, and worth experimenting with when cutting back on salt in cooking.

TASTY SAUCE TEMPLATE

The preparation used in the Savory Vegetables Template provides plenty of flavor. On occasion, however—or when you've simply prepared vegetables by steaming them—a tasty sauce like this one can provide the perfect finish.

3 cups cooked vegetables

¼ cup chopped onion, or 2 tablespoons dried onion flakes

1–2 tablespoons savory seasoning, to taste (ex: nutritional yeast, garlic powder, fresh dill, cilantro)

½–1 teaspoon salty seasoning, to taste (ex: miso paste, vegetable broth powder)

¼–½ cup plant milk or vegetable broth, as needed for desired thickness

1. Place the cooked vegetables, onion, seasonings, and a small amount of the plant milk in a food processor or blender. Process until the mixture reaches the desired consistency. Add more or less liquid or seasoning depending on your preference. Reheat in a saucepan if needed.

2. Top whole grains or baked potatoes with your vegetables of choice and ladle some of the warm sauce over all. Store leftovers in the refrigerator.

YIELD: About 2 cups

* * * * * **VARIATIONS** * * * * *

Prepare these variations following the same method as the Tasty Sauce Template (see above).

Tasty Sauce Template Variation #1: Creamy Corn Sauce

This adds a beautiful savory yet sweet golden crown to any vegetable, whole grain, or combination thereof.

3 cups or 1 (16-ounce) bag frozen corn, cooked

¼ cup chopped onion, or 2 tablespoons dried onion flakes

2 tablespoons nutritional yeast

1 teaspoon white miso paste

¼–½ cup plant milk or vegetable broth, as needed for desired thickness

NOTE

For a little extra zip, add 1 tablespoon white balsamic vinegar when processing the ingredients.

Tasty Sauce Template Variation #2: Bright Green Sauce

This sauce awakens the eye and taste buds with brilliant color—and is an easy way to sneak in more green!

    3 cups chopped broccoli or 1 (16-ounce) bag frozen peas, cooked
    ¼ cup chopped onion, or 2 tablespoons dried onion flakes
    2 tablespoons nutritional yeast
    1 teaspoon white miso paste
¼–½ cup plant milk or vegetable broth, as needed for desired thickness

BEAN SPREAD TEMPLATE

Bean spreads make quick and easy sandwich fillings, an irresistible dip for vegetables or baked chips, or, thinned with vinegar, a delicious dressing for salads, whole grains, or starchy vegetables.

   1   (15-ounce) can chickpea, pinto, or cannellini beans, rinsed and drained (about 1½ cups)

   1   tablespoon seed or nut butter, or ¼ cup pitted olives

1½   teaspoons seasonings, to taste (ex: cumin, paprika, chipotle)

   2   cloves garlic, crushed, or ¼ teaspoon garlic powder

  ¼   teaspoon mild yellow miso or salt, or ½ teaspoon tamari

   3   tablespoons lemon or lime juice

   2   tablespoons water, as needed

1. Place the ingredients except for the water in a food processor or blender. Process, adding the water 1 tablespoon at a time, to the desired texture (chunky or smooth).

YIELD: About 1 cup

NOTE

For a lower-fat version, eliminate the nut butter/olives; for a richer version, add more. Adjust the lemon/lime juice and garlic to taste. This goes fast, so I usually double the recipe.

* * * * * **VARIATIONS** * * * * *

Prepare these variations following the same method as the Bean Spread Template (see above).

Bean Spread Template Variation #1: Hummus

When nudging the oils out of your diet, mayo on sandwiches is an easy item to replace. Try using hummus instead. It's the new mayo!

   1   (15-ounce) can chickpeas, rinsed and drained (about 1½ cups)

   1   tablespoon tahini

   2   cloves garlic, crushed, or ¼ teaspoon garlic powder

  ½   teaspoon ground cumin

  ½   teaspoon ground coriander

  ¼   teaspoon mild yellow miso or salt, or 1 teaspoon tamari

3 tablespoons lemon juice
2 tablespoons water, as needed

NOTE

I like my hummus chunky, with big bits of chickpeas mixed in. To achieve this, process half of the chickpeas with the other ingredients to make a smooth paste, then use the "pulse" feature on the food processor or a potato masher to mix in the rest of the beans. You can also switch up the flavor of hummus by adding, during processing, a roasted red pepper, a handful of chopped cilantro or parsley, or a teaspoon of lemon zest.

Bean Spread Template Variation #2: Black Bean Chipotle

Black beans, chipotle, and adobo are a flavor match made in heaven. Try this recipe as veggie dip, as a sandwich spread, or simply rolled up in tortillas. The adobo kicks the heat in quickly—add to taste!

1 (15-ounce) can black beans, rinsed and drained (about 1½ cups)
½ cup pitted black olives
½ teaspoon ground cumin
½ teaspoon chipotle powder
½ teaspoon adobo
2 cloves garlic, crushed, or ¼ teaspoon garlic powder
2 tablespoons lime juice
½ teaspoon tamari
2 tablespoons water, as needed

COLOR AND CRUNCH SALAD TEMPLATE

This recipe simply combines colorful veggies in a quick, crisp salad.

> 3 cups crisp vegetables
> 1 cup greens
>   Oil-free salad dressing, lemon or lime juice, or vinegar, to taste

1. Toss the vegetables in a food processor for fast prep, or use any grating tool or knife to slice and shred the vegetables by hand. Tear the greens into bite-size pieces and combine with the vegetables in a large bowl.

2. Drizzle with the dressing and serve. Try topping with Lime Chipotle Chickpeas (page 206) or sunflower seeds lightly toasted in a skillet on the stove top.

YIELD: 2 large or 4 small salads

* * * * * **VARIATIONS** * * * * *

The combination options for this salad are only limited by the collection of crunchy roots, stems, and other plants that you have on hand. Simply chop the vegetables, drizzle with dressing of your choice, and serve!

Color and Crunch Salad Template Variation #1: Four Colors Crunch

With its orange, green, purple, and red, this salad is enchantment for the eye.

> 2 carrots, grated
> 1 cup sugar snap peas, chopped
> ½ purple onion, diced
> ½ red bell pepper, diced
> ¼ head green cabbage, grated or shredded
> ½ cup arugula, coarsely chopped

Color and Crunch Salad Template Variation #2: Purple Plus

According to a survey of eating and health habits conducted by the National Health and Nutrition Examination Study (NHANES), adults who eat purple and blue plants have reduced risk for high blood pressure and better levels of HDL cholesterol (the "good" kind). They are also less likely to be overweight. The compounds that give purple foods their color mop up free radicals and soothe inflammation. Currently, purple and blue foods make up only 3 percent of the average American's fruit and vegetable intake;[1] here's your opportunity to eat more.

    3 carrots, grated
    ½ head purple cabbage, shredded
    ½ sweet red onion, finely chopped

Color and Crunch Salad Template Variation #3: Crispy Potato

Here's the ultimate in salad crunch, with cooked potatoes as a smooth backdrop.

    2 carrots, shredded
    ½ jicama, shredded or chopped
    2 stalks celery, sliced
    2 cooked potatoes, cold, diced
    1 red bell pepper, seeded and chopped
    ½ cup cilantro, chopped, for garnish

PLANT BURGER TEMPLATE

Savory and satisfying, and loaded onto a whole grain bun with the works, a good burger is always a hit. Plant burgers—aka veggie burgers—are a popular transition food to carry well on into full-fledged practice of your plant-centered meals. I also affectionately call this variation of Plant Burgers the World Burger because I have made these all over the world using beans, grains, and vegetables found in local markets. The recipe template is drawn from the meat loaf formula Mom used when I was a kid: ground meat, chopped onions, tomato sauce for moisture, seasonings, and oatmeal or bread crumbs to bind it all together. I simply switched in meaty beans and grains (according to the dictionary, "meat" is the edible part of anything), added a variety of vegetables and seasonings, and dressed it in a nice crisp coating. This is a perfect example of taking a meal you already know and plantifying it.

Plant Burgers don't need to be limited to being served "burger style," either. I've used these same variations to create "meatballs" and served them with pasta or rice with a sauce, or broken them into bite-size croquettes to top a Buddha Bowl (page 112). Extremely versatile, these can be cooked up on the spot, or baked in batches to keep in the fridge or freezer for grabbing on the go.

BASE

    1 (15-ounce) can beans, rinsed and drained (about 1½ cups)

    1 cup cooked short-grain brown rice (see note)

VEGETABLES/NUTS

  1½ cups cut-up raw veggies (ex: ½ cup each of onions, carrots, and mushrooms, or any desired combination)

   ¼ cup chopped nuts (ex: walnuts, almonds, pine nuts) (optional; see note)

BINDER

    1 cup quick-cooking oatmeal or bread crumbs

SEASONINGS

    2 cloves garlic, crushed, or ½ teaspoon garlic powder

 1–2 tablespoons preferred spices and seasonings, to taste

   ½ teaspoon salt

MOISTENER

 2–3 tablespoons plant milk or vegetable broth, as needed

CRISP COATING

   ¼ cup cornmeal or garbanzo flour (more as needed)

1. Lightly pulse the beans in food processor, leaving some of the beans in chunks for texture, or partially mash with potato masher. Add to a large bowl along with the rice.

2. Finely chop the raw vegetables. I use my food processor, first cutting veggies into 1-inch pieces and then pulse using the "S" blade until finely chopped. Add the vegetables and nuts to the bowl with the beans and rice.

3. Add the binder and seasonings to the bowl and knead to make the mixture workable for forming burgers. Add the moistener, 1 tablespoon at a time, if it doesn't hold together well. Chill for an hour or more, if time allows.

4. Form the mixture into palm-size patties about ⅜ inch thick.

5. Place the coating on a plate. Lightly dust both sides of each burger, one at a time, by setting them gently onto the plate of coating. Roll the edges against a flat surface to make a round shape with flat sides and pat the coating onto the sides as well. This adds a nice crispy surface and helps the burgers keep their shape.

6. Cook in a nonstick pan over medium heat for 5 minutes, then turn and cook on the other side for an additional 4–5 minutes. You can also place on a baking sheet and bake at 350 degrees for about 20 minutes.

7. Serve on buns or alone with your favorite condiments. Expect a savory, soft texture in a thin, crisp crust.

YIELD: 7 or 8 palm-size burgers

NOTES

RICE NOTE: Short-grain brown rice has sticky properties that hold the burger together; substituting long-grain rice or another grain may result in a burger that falls apart more easily. For a more savory flavor, cook the rice in vegetable broth instead of water.

NUTS NOTE: While the nuts add texture and flavor, you can eliminate to reduce fat content.

✳ ✳ ✳ ✳ ✳ VARIATIONS ✳ ✳ ✳ ✳ ✳

Mix things up using different beans, grains, vegetables, and seasonings. Ingredients are organized by the role they play in the burger. Here are some variations. May it inspire your own flavor creations!

Prepare as in the Plant Burger Template (page 107).

Plant Burger Template Variation #1: Indian

This is my personal favorite Plant Burger variation, having gotten hooked on anything Indian food–related during my first travels to India.

BASE
- 1 (15-ounce) can chickpeas, rinsed and drained (about 1½ cups)
- 1 cup cooked short-grain brown rice

VEGETABLES/NUTS
- ½ cup chopped sweet onion
- ½ cup grated carrot
- ½ cup chopped baked potato
- ¼ cup chopped walnuts

BINDER
- 1 cup bread crumbs

SEASONINGS
- 1 clove garlic, crushed, or ½ teaspoon garlic powder
- 2 teaspoons curry vindaloo powder
- 1 teaspoon ground coriander
- ½ teaspoon salt

MOISTENER
- 2–3 tablespoons plant milk

CRISP COATING
- ¼ cup cornmeal or garbanzo flour (more as needed)

Plant Burger Template Variation #2: All-American

Try serving with sliced tomatoes, sweet onions, ketchup, mustard, barbecue sauce, and pickles or relish!

BASE
- 1 (15-ounce) can pinto beans, rinsed and drained (about 1½ cups)
- 1 cup cooked short-grain brown rice

VEGETABLES/NUTS
- ½ cup grated carrot
- ½ cup chopped onion
- ½ cup chopped mushrooms
- ¼ cup chopped walnuts

BINDER
- 1 cup quick-cooking oatmeal or bread crumbs

SEASONINGS
  1 clove garlic, crushed, or ½ teaspoon garlic powder
  1 tablespoon vegetarian Worcestershire sauce
  2 tablespoons nutritional yeast
  1 tablespoon chopped fresh dill, or 1 teaspoon dried
  2 teaspoons smoked paprika
  ¼ teaspoon liquid smoke

MOISTENER
  2–3 tablespoons ketchup or barbecue sauce

CRISP COATING
  ¼ cup cornmeal or garbanzo flour (more as needed)

Plant Burger Template Variation #3: Mexican

Try serving with avocado, tomato slices, and salsa.

BASE
  1 (15-ounce) can pinto or black beans, rinsed and drained (about 1½
     cups)
  1 cup cooked short-grain brown rice

VEGETABLES
  1½ cups total (in any combination) canned green chilies (drained),
      corn, onion, black olives, cilantro

BINDER
  1 cup quick-cooking oatmeal or bread crumbs

SEASONINGS
  1 teaspoon garlic powder
  2 teaspoons ground cumin
  2 teaspoons chili powder
  1 teaspoon chipotle powder
  ½–1 teaspoon red pepper flakes (if you like it hot!)

MOISTENER
  2–3 tablespoons salsa, as needed

CRISP COATING
  ¼ cup cornmeal or garbanzo flour (more as needed)

Plant Burger Deluxe: Smoky Black Bean Tempeh Burger

*An expanded version of the Plant Burger Template (page 107), this
burger has been specifically mentioned as being a huge hit from the*

beginning with families in transition to plant-based eating. You'll notice its template qualities, though it is listed here as a recipe because it is a bit more complex.

   1   (15-ounce) can black beans, rinsed and drained (about 1½ cups)

   1   large baked sweet potato

1¼   cups cooked short-grain brown rice

   4   ounces tempeh (if unable to find, use firm tofu instead)

  ¼   cup ketchup

   1   teaspoon garlic powder

   1   teaspoon tamari

   1   teaspoon vinegar (any kind)

  ¼   cup nutritional yeast

   1   teaspoon smoked paprika

       Splash of plant milk

BUDDHA BOWL TEMPLATE

This one-bowl meal connects the Easy Meal Planner with quick meal preparation into one delightful creation. Though there is no global agreement about what officially constitutes a Buddha bowl, what everyone does seem to agree upon is that they are universally satisfying and easy to pull together. Simple or complex as you like, highly portable and extremely flexible, Buddha bowls can be easily made in the workplace—simply pack separate containers with the layers ready to go and assemble on site.

Here is the basic construct of the infamous Buddha bowl. All measurements are approximate—go with your mood.

> 2 handfuls leafy greens (ex: kale, spinach, romaine, arugula)
>
> 1½ cups cooked whole grains or pasta, warm or cold
>
> 1½ cups chopped raw or cooked vegetables or fruit in any combination (ex: yams, squash, beets, broccoli, carrots, roasted eggplant, apples)
>
> ½ cup beans, legumes, tofu, or tempeh

1. Heap all the ingredients—warm, cold, or a combination—into a large bowl of your choice, or assemble side by side on a plate.

2. Top with sauce or dressing of your choice (see page 202 for ideas).

YIELD: 1 bowl

* * * * * VARIATIONS * * * * *

Prepare these variations following the same method as the Buddha Bowl Template (see above).

Buddha Bowl Template Variation #1: Middle Eastern

For dressing, try topping with Tahini-Lemon Sauce (page 202), Sweet and Sour Dressing (page 202), or thin Hummus (page 103) with vinegar to desired consistency.

> 2 handfuls torn romaine lettuce
>
> 1½ cups cooked bulgur wheat
>
> 1½ cups chopped cucumber, tomatoes, diced red onion, grated carrot, and finely chopped parsley in any combination
>
> ½ cup Hummus or chickpeas

Buddha Bowl Template Variation #2: Mexican

Try using ½ cup tomato salsa as dressing!

   2 handfuls baby spinach leaves

1½ cups cooked brown rice

1½ cups cubed cooked zucchini, chopped tomatoes, grated jicama,
      diced sweet onion, and finely chopped cilantro in any combination

  ½ cup black beans

Buddha Bowl Template Variation #3: African

On safari in Africa might be the last place you'd expect to find plenty of good plant-based options. Yet that's exactly what my husband, Greg, and I found—every meal there was a smorgasbord of choices for building bowls just like this one. Vegetables and ugali—African polenta—were served at every meal.

Try topping with Mbegu's Spicy African Peanut Sauce (page 203).

   2 handfuls baby spinach and/or baby kale

1½ cups ugali or polenta, cooked as for Black Bean Polenta Pie (page 192)
      or according to package instructions

1½ cups shredded carrot, chopped tomatoes, chopped sweet onion,
      and kale cooked Savory Vegetables style in any combination

  ½ cup cooked lentils

SIMPLE VEGETABLE SOUP TEMPLATE

This is my original five-ingredient recipe. There are several ways to vary the outcome depending on the variety of lentils (red, orange, green), the greens you put in the pot, and the selection of root vegetables that you use. I also call this "Triple S Soup" because it is simple, satisfying, and slimming.

1 **cup lentils, soaked overnight (see note)**

3 **large root vegetables (ex: carrots, potatoes)**

2 **large onions, coarsely chopped**

1 **large bunch dark leafy greens (ex: kale, chard, spinach)**

½ **cup dried shiitake mushrooms (you can also use fresh or canned—dried shiitakes have a stronger flavor)**

Vegetable bouillon, miso paste, salt, or other soup seasoning and spices to taste

1. Put about 3 inches of water in a pressure cooker and place on high heat.

2. Add the soaked lentils, bring to a boil, and cook for 10 minutes.

3. Coarsely chop the root vegetables—I slice them in the food processor to make it fast and easy. Add the vegetables and onions to the lentils. Add water as needed to rise 2 to 3 inches over the top of the lentils and vegetables.

4. Tear or chop dark leafy greens into bite-size pieces and add to the lentil and vegetable mixture along with the mushrooms. Cook at pressure for 3 to 4 minutes. Release the pressure, then stir and season the soup as you wish with vegetable bouillon, miso paste, or other soup seasoning and spices. Serve.

YIELD: 4 servings

NOTES

LENTIL NOTE: If you don't soak the lentils in advance, you'll have to add a little cooking time. If using tiny orange lentils, there's no need to soak them.

NOTE: This soup can also be made in a slow cooker or on the stove top without a pressure cooker—it just takes a little longer.

✳ ✳ ✳ ✳ ✳ VARIATION ✳ ✳ ✳ ✳ ✳

Prepare this variation following the same method as the Simple Vegetable Soup Template (page 114).

Simple Vegetable Soup Template
Variation: French Green Lentil Soup

French green lentils hold their shape more than other varieties, and the celery adds a distinctive flavor to this variation.

2 large sweet potatoes, cut into chunks
2 large white onions, chopped
1 cup French green lentils, soaked overnight
1 large bunch purple kale
1 cup chopped celery
   Vegetable bouillon, miso paste, salt, or other soup seasoning and spices to taste (add after cooking)

FRUIT MOUSSE TEMPLATE

When something a little more fancy is called for, this can be just the ticket—a sweet winner with kids and grown-ups alike. Sprinkle with chocolate nibs or carob powder for an extra treat.

> 2 cups chopped frozen fruit
> 1 cup plant milk
> 1 teaspoon vanilla bean paste or vanilla extract

1. Place the fruit in the food processor or blender with 2–3 tablespoons of the plant milk and vanilla bean paste or extract and start to blend.

2. Add plant milk 1 tablespoon at a time as you continue to tamp the mousse down to keep it thick yet moving.

3. Scoop into bowls and serve with a spoon.

YIELD: 2 servings

NOTE

You need a pretty robust blender to make Fruit Mousse because it demands brute strength of the blending blade and motor. I use my food processor, though I know there are other blenders that are up to the task!

* * * * * **VARIATIONS** * * * * *

Prepare these variations following the same method as the Fruit Mousse Template (see above).

Fruit Mousse Template Variation #1: Chocolate Cherry Mousse

With a flavor reminiscent of chocolate-covered cherries, this variation is rich and sweet.

> 2 cups pitted frozen cherries
> 1 teaspoon vanilla bean paste or vanilla extract
> 1 cup almond milk
> 2 tablespoons cocoa or carob powder

Fruit Mousse Template Variation #2: Blueberry Date Mousse

The dates sweeten any tartness from the blueberries in this beautifully colored version.

2   cups frozen blueberries

1   teaspoon vanilla bean paste or vanilla extract

1   cup almond milk

3   dates, soaked

ROCK STAR

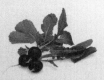

*Taking Plant-Based Eating to a
Bigger Stage: Handling Work, Travel,
and Family and Friends*

CHAPTER 9
Plant-Based on the Road

You may be experiencing a few lingering challenges when it comes to plant-based eating. Each has the potential to slow down the ride to realizing your health, weight, or lifestyle ideal. Maybe you are having trouble being prepared when you step outside the convenience of home. Or possibly you're finding it hard to let go of those last edible holdouts that aren't in alignment with your new plan. First, we'll focus on how to take what's become easy at home—the systems you've rooted yourself in as Rookie—and transfer them to workplace readiness. From there, we'll address travel, so that you can easily take living plant-based everywhere.

Acknowledge the successes and powerful shifts you have already made. At this stage of the journey, plenty of substantial fare is showing up on your plate in the form of big scoops of beans, starchy vegetables, and whole grains. You are easily eating seven or more helpings of nonstarchy vegetables and fruits each day. You may be enjoying more of one and less of the other—and that's as it should be, for we each have to find our own personal meal mojo. You may well already find yourself fully immersed in plant-based living. If so, the Ten-Day Plant-Based Makeover coming up in chapter 11 looks just like how you eat day-to-day now. Stars all over the chart!

Even if all is well and good when it comes to being prepared with plenty of healthful eats at home, the leap to taking plant-based outside the front door can be baffling. For some, this comes easily. Yet if making this maneuver hasn't come readily for you, you are not alone. This chapter will help you tackle eating outside of your home.

HOW TO SYSTEMATIZE WORKPLACE READINESS

Putting systems in place for workplace readiness is one of the most common circumstances with which people need assistance in the plant-based transition. I speak from experience on this one as well. For twenty years, I taught middle school full-time. In addition, several evenings a week, I was teaching classes at college and university. This translated into ten- to twelve-hour workdays, including commute time and squeezing in my own workouts. Somehow, I also had to make sure my kitchen and workplace were stocked with the food I needed. This meant building systems to make it work. I found I could multiply the joy and benefits of living plant-based by keeping priorities: simplicity, planning, and preparation. The rewards, I found—as will you—are enormous.

With a 7:00 A.M. liftoff time each morning for my commute, it meant I had to get an early start on being ready with food packed to take with me for the day. With only twenty to twenty-five minutes for lunch—I didn't have the luxury of eating out—that meant fitting out my food bag to go the daily distance. This involved several containers packed with salads, sandwiches, fruit, vegetables, and leftovers. I purchased a small refrigerator to keep near my desk area in the classroom so that good plant eats were within easy reach. In addition to what I brought each day for my meals, I kept this refrigerator stocked with fruit, vegetables such as carrots, celery, and sugar snap peas, and good grainy bread. In other words, I left nothing to chance, decreasing the odds that I'd fall face-first into any of those interesting edibles ubiquitous in the staff room.

Did I ever grumble and complain about taking the time to prepare each morning? You bet. Finally I figured out that getting food ready the night before was the solution, saving me the hectic push in the morning. It still took time to accomplish. But whenever I started whining about the inconvenience of having to get food ready to go, I would remind myself that it was far less inconvenient than being fat and hungry at the same time.

Preparation and simplicity—your watchwords for getting started as Rookie—are just as important when it comes to the workplace. Use this systems checklist to keep yourself plant-prepared.

Assess Your Food Needs for the Week Ahead

Before you grocery shop, mentally walk through the week ahead and acknowledge each time you are going to need to be prepared with food. That means every meal and every eating event anticipated—at home and away. Consider the unpredictable as well.

You needn't plan a special recipe for each lunch or dinner, unless this helps. Think from the Easy Meal Planner and recipe templates perspective. You know that for dinner each night you'll need a vegetable or two, a whole grain or starchy vegetable, probably beans or legumes, and quite likely some salad. For every lunch you'll need the same—it just might look a little different if it needs to be mobile. And if each of these categories doesn't make it to each meal—which happens, and doesn't really matter—at least you are prepared.

Build Your Market List

From there, build your shopping list. Keep a running list in the kitchen during the week as things come up so that you aren't starting from scratch as you pull into the parking lot at the market. Soon you'll develop a roster of favorites and regulars that you can organize into a checklist to make it easier. Utilize the shopping list in the appendix (page 216) to assist you. Giving yourself lead time with list building before you get to the market is a critical part of being prepared and an important way of supporting yourself. Buy and prepare more food than you think you'll need.

Pack and Take Food with You

If you're hungry, you're at work, and your food is at home, it's no good to you. You can't eat what you don't have. Conversely, what you have is what you'll eat—and that means whatever happens to find its way in front of you. And we know what that can mean. Don't leave it to chance. Unless you have a nearby healthy alternative, food will need to be brought with you from home in portable and durable containers. This is also the perfect venue for leftovers.

An easy solution for lunch is to pack sandwiches of Hummus (page 103) or other bean spread on whole grain bread or tortillas. Pack leftover Savory Vegetables (page 99) served over rice, quinoa, potatoes, or yams snatched from that big batch you cooked Sunday afternoon. If you have no idea where you'll be when midday hunger hits, or frequently find yourself far from food when you most need it, plan for it. You can pick up an insulated food bag—many department stores now carry these as stylish, gender-neutral shoulder bags. These can also be ordered online and will keep your food fresher for the day in the event you can't count on a fridge or cooler for storage. Pack items as suggested above, or simply fill your bag with cold baked potatoes or yams, fruit such as apples, oranges, mandarins, or bananas, durable easy-to-eat vegetables such as carrots and sugar snap peas, and toss in a hearty veggie wrap or Speedy Burrito (page 200). Fitted out like this, you'll even be able to parade your portable food right into the movie theater and the ticket-taker won't bat an eye. Speaking from experience.

Stock the Fridge at Work

To support your food plan for the week, think ahead with quantity cooking for work just as you do at home. Prepare a pot of plain brown rice or Golden Turmeric Rice (page 195) and bring in a big stack of Plant Burgers (page 107) to keep in the office fridge or freezer. Take in a big container of Game-Changer Chili (page 193) or simply cook a stash of black beans that will last a few days. What about picking up a few bags of ready-to-go greens for salads while you are at it? Stock a cupboard with plant-based dry soup mixes. Keep silverware and a big bowl or plate ready to fill with eats at your workplace. This means when its lunchtime, all you need to do is heap salad vegetables in a bowl and scoop some rice and beans over the top, Buddha Bowl (page 112) style. With simple salad dressing at hand, along with containers of salsa or other favorite toppings—covered if you've got the chili (and perhaps some Country Comfort Corn Bread on page 194)—don't be surprised if your coworkers start coveting your meals.

Stock Your Car

If your work schedule finds you frequently on the road, a cooler for your car is an important investment. Stock it with food for the day and keep it supplied with backup stash in the form of fruits, raw vegetables, baked potatoes, and some good grainy bread. Dried fruits and nuts are durable as second backup in your desk, car, or bag.

RESTAURANT TIPS

The workplace and travel both bring up the question of restaurant dining. Restaurant menus, it seems, are designed to thwart your best-laid plans for healthy eating. Oil, butter, and cheese are slammed into everything imaginable to increase food seduction, pushing you to keep eating. Is it any wonder Julia Child's cookbooks are such big sellers? Put gobs of butter in anything and it will taste good. When it comes to restaurant menus, here are a few simple strategies for navigating the options.

How to Put a Restaurant Plate Together

Restaurants listed as vegetarian, vegan, or natural foods may be friendly houses of food for your journey—but then again, perhaps not. Vegetarian implies no meat products; vegan items are devoid of all animal products. "Vegetarian" and "vegan," however, do not necessarily mean "healthy." They don't tell you anything about how the food is prepared, how much fat or sugar is added to the fare, or—in the case of vegetarian—even if dairy products or eggs are used. That doesn't mean these restaurant venues aren't workable; it just means that you will need to be specific about exactly what you want when ordering.

The best strategy is to do an internet search on the restaurant's menu—and even make a phone call in advance to inquire about options. Detect which items on the menu might be most plant-eater friendly. Most restaurants have a dinner salad on the menu. When ordering your salad, clearly underscore what you *do* want: lettuce, tomatoes, carrots, cucumber—any and all raw vegetables. Next, politely be specific about what you do *not* want on your salad—cheese, eggs, bacon, meat chunks, anchovies—I've been surprised by every one of these on one occasion or another. Don't be afraid to use the words "allergy" or "doctor" if it will help. Mention "no croutons" as well—they are usually fried in oil and often cheese saturated. Finally, ask for dressing on the side. You can also say "no dressing" and ask for a shaker of vinegar, which many restaurants serve with salads. With practice, you'll get better and better at asking for what you want. The waitstaff is there to serve you. Yet being especially courteous, appreciative, and friendly will make menu adjustments the best experience for everyone involved. You want the waiter or waitress to be your friend, and as you are asking them to go out of their way a bit for you, being gracious is a smart move.

More and more often, veggie burgers are being featured as sandwich or entrée menu choices. Ask that yours be baked and not fried, and ask for ketchup and mustard instead of mayo or butter on the bun. If there is a vegetarian sandwich listed, simply ask that yours be served without mayo, cheese, or butter. If not, you can probably order a custom sandwich.

In addition to salads and veggie burgers, your best restaurant bet might be in the sides section of the menu, where you will often find baked potatoes and other vegetables. If you don't see it listed, ask about the vegetable of the day, often served with the restaurant entrées as part of the main menu—frequently asparagus, green beans, or broccoli. You can ask that your serving be steamed and prepared without frying or oily dressing. If you say "low fat," all bets are off as to how butter-drenched your plate will arrive, so be specific. Fruit salads are usually either in the sides or listed somewhere else on the menu; clarify to serve without yogurt or cheese. Breakfast is usually easy because oatmeal is almost always on the menu. I've started to have increasing good luck with asking for soy milk or almond milk on the side, too.

Our recent stop at a Mexican eatery is an example of getting good choices at restaurants. On the face of it, the menu looked like a dietary disaster. But I know I can pull together something pretty good at most Mexican restaurants—as long as they have a batch of beans cooked sans lard. I had phoned ahead about the beans, so I knew that they had two pots of beans in the kitchen: one of them plain boiled pintos.

When we arrived, I knew exactly what to do. I ordered a big bowl of the boiled beans, a stack of soft, fresh corn tortillas, garden salad without dressing, extra bowls of salsa (for dressing and for my tacos), and some lime or lemon wedges. When it all arrived, I created multiple tacos by piling the beans, greens, and chunky house salsa on the corn tortillas. Combined with the greens and tomato on the salad, I crafted a hearty lunch. If the only in-house beans had been cooked in a pot of lard, I would have simply passed on beans in my tacos and done just fine with the fresh corn tortillas, tomatoes, green salad, and house salsa.

Big Chain Bites

When it comes to the fast-food chains, a little creativity can get you some eats in a pinch. The problem is all the mystery ingredients. Careful scrutiny usually uncovers dairy products, eggs, or oils on the lists of what, on the face of it, may appear to be plant-friendly fare—such as beans and veggie burgers. Ingredients seem to also be in a constant state of flux. You can't always trust that the servers are in the know when it comes to ingredients, so it's worth checking with management or headquarters online if you want to get the facts.

With so many fast-food establishments in the marketplace, there isn't room to do an exhaustive guide here. For now, here's a list of some of the most common establishments and options at each.

- **Arby's: Side salad, sans the cheese and croutons.**
- **Au Bon Pain: Sandwiches and salads, customized to not include animal products.**
- **Burger King: House salad with vinegar.**
- **Chipotle: Vegetarian burrito or bowl—their vegetarian beans have rice bran oil, so if you want to go oil-free you can construct a meal by ordering a veggie bowl and heap with lettuce, corn, salsa, tomato, peppers, guacamole, and vinegar.**
- **At Taco Bell, Chili's, and Baja Fresh, most items can be made with beans instead of meat, though their websites either list oils in the beans or rice or simply don't say. You can, however, easily avoid meat, cheese, and sour cream in burritos and bowls.**
- **Wendy's: Order from the salad bar with plain baked potatoes.**
- **Olive Garden: Go for a bottomless bowl of fresh salad—ask them to hold the cheese, dressing, and croutons, and serve vinegar on the side.**

The best resource I have found on fast-food restaurant menus is listed at Urban Tastebuds, which has ferreted out and listed "Forty-Eight Vegan Chain Restaurant Menus"—the closest thing to plant-based currently available. See the list at www.urbantastebuds.com/43-vegan-chain-restaurant-menus -every-vegan-needs-know. The list starts with Atlanta Bread Company and runs all the way through Wendy's. Each listing is linked to a page elaborating upon which items can be ordered without animal products. Keep in mind that it doesn't add the processed food filter, so items may include oils and other processed products. Fast-food meals are best left as last-resort options. Still, it's nice to know where you might be able to find emergency fare.

PLANES, TRAINS, AND AUTOMOBILES

What about the challenges posed by airplane and other long-distance travel? The tips regarding workplace readiness may be all you need. Yet travel involving greater distances and extended chunks of time presents its own set of challenges. This year my husband and I took five trips involving international travel. Add to that the dozen or so excursions made in country for speaking engagements, and we're talking about lots of hours logged on planes, in airports, and even a boat or two. The same pack-and-plan system works for all of them.

Scout the Location in Advance

The first thing I do for airplane travel is some reconnaissance regarding food options at the destination. First stop is the internet, where I'll search the hotel or rental location for nearby plant-food-friendly options, such as a produce market, a natural foods store, or a familiar chain—places where I've found a good meal in the past, and where I know I can replenish my travel food stash. I then search the area for restaurants under the categories of vegetarian, vegan, or natural foods. A search at www.happycow.net can often turn up several appropriate vendors for eats in urban areas.

Outbound

It's easy to prepare and pack food when you are heading out on plane travel. Here's an example of how I do it. With an international junket coming up in a few days from this writing—in addition to the in-transit needs of spare clothing and a toothbrush—I'll pack in my carry-on the following: four hummus sandwiches, two peanut butter sandwiches, four apples, cold baked potatoes, peeled carrots, sugar snap peas, and a couple of baggies of rolled oats along with some dried fruit, nuts, and seeds. All of these easily pass at airline security—I've never had a question asked yet. This food cache translates to two substantial meals for both my husband and me. The hummus sandwiches are eaten first due to their perishable nature. The carrots and snap peas will serve as filling and fibrous portable fare—instant salad, just not in the usual bowl. The peanut butter sandwiches pass the durability test and I've served them good as new— though slightly reshaped depending on the rigors of travel—up to forty-eight hours later. The apples last indefinitely. So do the nuts and seeds. Potatoes are best eaten within a few hours, depending on the heat to which your luggage is exposed, but I'm always impressed by the way these hold up. The rolled oats can be emptied into a cup, covered with water, and after a few minutes of soaking, ready to eat. If your fruit stockpile has run out, you can find apples, bananas, and other fruit at most airports, even in the coffee shops. Another option for carry-on is soups-in-a-cup that simply require hot water. Let them sit, and in five minutes you can have split pea or black bean soup.

Inbound

Returning from a destination creates a slightly different situation because you don't have the luxury of being able to stock up from home. If you've been staying with friends or family, a house rental, or a hotel with a fridge, you can pack fruit and durable sandwiches for the return trip. Rolled oats, dried fruit, and nuts packed as part of your outbound preparations can hitch up with airport salads and fruit for sustenance.

TAKING A PLANT-BASED STAND

Taking plant-based eating mainstream and into more and more eating establishments is a grassroots movement. It is growing stronger every day—increasing your dining-out options—simply because more and more of us are taking a stand with our forks at restaurants. It is precisely because those who have gone before you have asked for veggie burgers, oatmeal, and salad with vinegar on the side that these eats are easier and easier to find on restaurant menus, or ask for without raising an eyebrow. Continue the tradition and ease the way for those who follow you. Help grow the movement for more menu options by simply asking for what you want, which will return as a favor to you by giving you more options down the road.

When ordering in a restaurant, if what you want is not on the menu, politely ask for it, in person, over the phone, or both. For example, it's breakfast, and you order a bowl of oatmeal. Simply ask, "Do you have almond milk?" or "Do you have soy milk?" Even if you are not a big nondairy milk drinker, and you just like a splash on your early morning oats, stating the question brings the issue into the public eye. I can get by just fine without plant milk on my hot grains, yet sometimes I'll ask for it, if for no other reason than to send the message that plant-based replacements are now going mainstream.

Vendors respond to customer demand. Their desire is to please you so that you remain a loyal customer. Case in point: Recently finding ourselves on an island in Micronesia, my husband, Greg, and I stayed at a hotel that included a breakfast buffet. There was fruit, salad, bread—and then a long line of eggs, bacon, mystery meat stirred into some veggies, and of all things cocoa puffs and sugar-frosted flakes. We asked for soy milk and muesli, which we'd spotted in the public market down the street. Guess what the staff proudly presented us with the next morning? Don't apologize for what you eat. Ask for it!

Armed with multiple systems for workplace readiness, you may now be struggling with how to bring the family along. Next, we'll look at what may be challenging on the home front. You'll hear from several parents about how they've engineered the transition with their families—and from some of the kids as well.

CHAPTER 10
Family, Friends, and Food Pushers

Once you are ready for the workplace, travel, and busy schedule days, how can you bring the kids along? What about all the other venues to navigate where food seems to take center stage, such as family gatherings and other social situations? And how do you deal with food pushers, who were enough of a challenge before? This chapter will prepare you for all the social challenges you might encounter as you start eating plant-based.

BRINGING THE KIDS ALONG

Adopting a new food plan, for most of us, means figuring out how to make it work with the family. Ideally, your plant-based food plan will bring your family together, rather than resulting in tension and dissension. Yet as with any change, you can expect some growing pains. And if you are the sole source of plant-based inspiration for your family unit, conversations and negotiations with your partner may be in order so that you can implement a united approach when it comes to the kids.

Each family situation is different, yet the bottom line is this: If you are a parent, you are in the best place to influence the diet of your children. They learn by the behavior that you model—nothing new there. If you are removing animal products and processed foods from your diet, their plates will reflect yours. If you are positive, excited, and adventurous, their attitudes will mirror that, too.

> **MODELING CHOICES FOR YOUR CHILDREN**
>
> A recent study published in the *New England Journal of Medicine* shows that kids who are overweight in kindergarten are often condemned to future obesity.[1] You can best support the future health of your children by the choices you make—and model—for them now. "A plant-based diet seems to be a sensible approach for the prevention of obesity in children," states a 2013 Nutritional Update for Physicians in the *Permanente Journal.*[2]

Behavioral Economics

You may already know from experience that trying to force your kids to eat against their will can polarize the situation. If you've been frustrated in the past by trying to get your kids to eat this or that, take comfort—and insight—from what the research tells us. Requiring cafeteria students to eat vegetables had virtually no impact on vegetable consumption—it only doubled the waste from vegetables.[3] But what if the students were given the choice between two different vegetables?

In a recent experiment conducted at Cornell, 120 junior high students were told they must take carrots with their lunch, while another 120 were given the choice of carrots *or* celery. The idea was to discover whether giving children a choice over which vegetable to eat would increase the consumption of vegetables overall. This is called "provision of choice," a branch of behavioral economics. Of those required to take the carrots, 69 percent ate them, while 91 percent of those who had a choice between carrots or celery ate their vegetables.[4] These same results have been underscored in similar studies: Children given the "provision of choice" over which vegetable to eat at lunch granted them increased personal autonomy. Consumption of vegetables increased by as much as 80 percent.[5]

Does this mean that to get your kids to eat vegetables you have to give them multiple choices at each meal? Maybe. But a more practical yet effective idea is to grant your children some of the decision making about the dishes you prepare. For this reason, a parental approach that comes from authority—without being authoritarian—and gives children the empowerment of choice is what has proven most successful. You'll see this clearly illustrated in the three family stories featured later in this chapter. In addition to provision of choice, here are more suggestions to get you started in bringing your family with you on the plant-based journey.

Increase Food Variety

Maybe your children don't like peas or beets but take to green beans and sweet potatoes. Introducing different vegetables to them over the course of the week gives them a chance to learn which ones they like. And don't be afraid to revisit those initially passed over—kids' tastes change and what may not necessarily appeal one day might look inviting on another.

Offer Veggies Before Dinner

Providing a selection of celery, carrots, tomatoes, jicama, broccoli, and other fresh vegetables available with a dish of bean dip will meet the needs of kids eager for dinner. Hungry kids go for this big-time, and you don't have to worry about getting more veggies in later. In addition, roasting potatoes, carrots, peppers, squash, and even tomatoes gives the vegetables a different flavor that has proven to be kid-friendly.

Focus on the Positive and Make It Tasty

Children don't respond to the threat of disease as adults do—but they will respond to abundant, delicious food. Consider introducing the transition as an adventure in eating. Take your kids to the market with you to select grains, fruits, and vegetables. Farmers' markets are a playground of produce, and your children will have the opportunity to participate in the fun of choice. Then, once you're back home, involve them in food prep with their selections. Food that your kids can easily prepare and serve proudly wins their hearts and minds.

Plant a Vegetable Garden as a Family Project

The excitement of growing their own food is an irresistible enticement to try something new. Plus, you'll give your kids more autonomy with the power to "grow their own."

FROM THE HOME FRONT

Several responders to the Plant-Based Transitions Survey elaborated upon details of the family portion of the plant-based journey. As you'll see below, Sue, Amy, and Sharon engineered their family's food plan change in slightly different ways. Yet note the commonalities: parental leadership that shows up as clarity and consistency. You'll also hear from Sharon's three children who describe the family plant-based adventures from their perspective as kids, tweens, and teens. Rock Stars all.

"Determination and Planning Are Essential"

Busy mom and cycling enthusiast, Sue, along with her husband, started eating plant-based five years ago. Finding go-to meals and realizing early on that keeping it simple—utilizing the Easy Meal Planner concept—were keys to their success. "I still remember the initial days after making the decision to change our eating," Sue told me. "I struggled to create meals that were plant-based, not really understanding how to do this in a practical way for my own family. The recipes I found seemed to feature items as some sort of 'main dish.' Sure, I could make a bean casserole, but what about the traditional vegetable side dish—like the frozen peas and carrots I used to serve? Would I offer this alongside the bean casserole? How would it look on the plate? I thought that the fancier the recipe, the more my family would like it. In hindsight, however, I realize that I made the transition to plant-based eating far more difficult than it needed to be."

Sue shared that the first two days were the hardest for her teenagers. Familiar foods were missed, and new flavors and textures were not immediately liked. She quickly learned that the best way to invite family cooperation is to create simple yet delicious, satisfying meals—for tastelessness is the fastest track to dissidence. "Surprisingly, by the third day—and, after realizing that there would be nothing else served but the new, healthier food—everyone began to like the meals," she explained. "I had two or three recipes that I cooked over and over again until I figured out what I was doing, and it wasn't long before we found a week's worth of recipes that we all liked and that were quick to prepare."

Sue understood that having her entire family on board with the change made the transition much easier. If you are not experiencing family solidarity, however, sometimes it is easier to transition into healthier eating gradually. Sue shared: "I have a friend whose husband and children are the 'meat and potatoes' types, but they have started eating several meatless meals a week. Another friend is learning how to prepare meals for her family that will incorporate her own health goals by substituting meat—prepared for them—with starches, whole grains, legumes, and vegetables—for her. Many recipes or meal plans can be made to overlap two ways of eating. It isn't always easy, but the extra effort is better than giving up one's desire to get healthy. One of the biggest challenges that women in particular face is when they are the only one in their family who has the desire to make a diet change. It can be very hard to stay on course when you feel you are alone on the journey, so I encourage everyone to surround themselves with information, recipe ideas, and others who share similar interests."

Sue sums it up like this: "The meals I cook for my family are simple, yet healthful and filling. I always keep these staples on hand: cooked brown rice, cooked sweet and white potatoes, canned beans, and fresh and frozen vegetables. Over the years I've come to understand that determination and planning are essential. We love our new way of eating. Not only do we feel it is best for our health, but we have also come to appreciate how it is friendlier to the world around us—the environment, animals, and people in poorer countries. We tell anyone who asks us about the changes they have seen in our own lives to try this way of eating for themselves. They have nothing to lose and much to gain. A plant-based diet goes a long way toward making life better."

Pantry Purge, a Year-Long Commitment—and Bringing Four Kids Along

Amy Montoya's plant-based journey was precipitated by a health crisis, inspiring her to jump the family all the way into plant-based overnight. "I had been very sick for over a year, at one point completely bedridden for several months," said Amy. "I just wanted to feel better and heal my body. I had dealt with weight problems my whole life, but never really health problems. I was desperate to try anything to help me become healthy again. My dad brought over a plant-based nutrition book, saying it just might help me. I read the book that night, then went out and bought *The China Study* to learn more about the science behind it. When my husband came home from work the next day, I announced that we were now eating all plant-based!"

Amy continued: "I believed in it and committed to doing it for one full year and seeing what happened." She gave away every food in their pantry, fridge, freezer, and storage room that was not on the plan. Amy and her husband made commitments to each other that they would not buy any food off the plant-based plan for one full year. "It was very hard for about three weeks. The kids were having a hard time at first, but when they got hungry, they ate! I wanted the results promised by eating a whole food–based diet and knew I couldn't say it failed or didn't work if I didn't do it 100 percent. We have been to birthday parties, family celebrations, and holiday events and we have said the kids can eat whatever they want because we do not have anything at home that is off plan—ever. The kids know the house rules and they live by them—they don't fight them at all. When and if we go out to eat, we only get plant-based items. If we—as their parents—are convinced and committed, it is not a debate."

Amy's family has been whole food plant-exclusive now for one year. The kids were nineteen, six, four, and two years old at the time they started. Reports Amy, "The whole family is on board. I am off every med and down 46 pounds, and my total cholesterol is 113. My husband has lost about 30 pounds and his cholesterol is down from 273 to 192. We also had huge improvements in our A1Cs—an important blood test used to determine how well diabetes is being controlled—blood pressures, fasting blood glucose, and all our lipid panels. No turning back—this is our life and we love it." Here are some of Amy's top tips for family success.

Create a Food-Safe Environment

This is the greatest factor for bringing the children along. If you have junk foods, processed foods, meats, or cheeses, they will want to eat them. They'll be confused and fight you at mealtimes. But if they can open the fridge or pantry and know that anything in there is good to eat, they will eat it when they are hungry.

Everyone Eats the Same Food

Sit down, eat as one, and enjoy the new foods together. Amy's rule is "you don't have to like everything but you do need to eat it for this one meal."

Find What You Like and What Your Family Likes; Plan and Prepare

Choose whole foods and vegetables you already love and then just add to them. Find a few recipes your family already likes and make them plant-based so you can enjoy the transition.

Lead by Example

It is not fair to the children to see you "cheating" on foods that don't nourish your body and then refuse to give it to them when they ask—and they *will* ask.

Keep It Simple

It doesn't have to be fancy—just healthy and tasty. Amy's family favorite go-tos are simple meals such as bean burritos, lentil tacos, spaghetti, chili, soups and stews, plant burgers with oven fries, stir-fries, and veggie pizza— all with salads or cooked vegetables on the side. Invest in a pressure cooker; it really helps with time management. And eating this way is not expensive.

Cherish the Time It Takes to Succeed and Think of It as a Gift to Yourself and Your Family

Have fun, experiment, and enjoy your food. You don't have to eat this specific vegetable or spice or buy "superfoods." Cheese was the hardest thing for Amy's family to give up—and baked chips were the hardest food for her to give up, but now she makes her own! You do go through taste changes, but if you delay it you are always fighting it. Once you make the shift, all you do is reap the results.

The McRae Family: How Sharon Transitioned Her Family to a Plant-Based Plate

Health coach and cooking instructor Sharon McRae, and her husband, Dave, a practicing lawyer, live in Maryland with their three children. Full of insights and practical strategies for family change, here is the story of Sharon's plant-based journey, and how she brought her family along with her. Immediately following, you'll hear from the McRae kids—Tess, Marcie, and Evan—reporting in from their unique perspective.

"I'm the mom of three very unusual kids," Sharon began, "or so I'm told. To me, they're pretty typical. They love to play computer games, hate to go to bed, and now that my twin daughters are in high school, there's a lot of eye rolling, and lots of silliness and roughhousing from my younger son. The way in which they are unusual has everything to do with what they are eating. Though raised vegetarians, until five years ago, they ate lots of dairy-based foods like pizza, macaroni and cheese, and ice cream, as well as lots of processed vegetarian foods. That all changed the day I sat them down and told them, 'No more dairy!' They all cried—but fast-forward five years. Now they all happily enjoy healthy delights like roasted Brussels sprouts, cheesy kale chips, and black bean brownies.

"My personal transition to a completely plant-based diet was gradual. In my late teens, I made the connection between the roast beef that was on my plate and the cows that were on the TV on the newscast one night, and I decided I could no longer eat red meat. I stopped eating poultry in my twenties, when as a biology major in college I couldn't help myself from dissecting my KFC dinner. Seafood went in my thirties, when I was pregnant and concerned about mercury levels. From that time on, I was eating a vegetarian diet, though one heavy in the fake meats, dairy, and eggs.

"We lost my mom to cancer in April 2009. She had gotten the initial diagnosis years before, which caused me to make some major changes in my own lifestyle. It wasn't until the end stages of her life—when I was spending long days in the cancer ward at Johns Hopkins Hospital—that a voice inside me told me to stop eating animal protein. I decided to give it a go—no more animal products for two weeks, without telling anyone else—and see how I did.

"The two weeks passed, and I realized I felt better without eating dairy products. I 'came out' to my family. Everyone panicked. The kids cried, fearful this would mean a change for them because they really loved their dairy products. I reassured everyone that this was just something that I was doing—I wasn't going to change anything for anyone else.

"Shortly after my mom died, I decided to start a new career as a health coach. I read *The China Study*, which opened my eyes to the terrible health consequences of including animal protein in your diet. I explained to the kids in clear terms why we were making this transition. They all cried again—real tears. They were terrified about losing their favorite foods. I reassured them that I would make it easy for them and that I was doing this out of love for them. I found a nondairy 'cheese' that they really loved, and with it I continued to prepare their favorite comfort foods: pizza, macaroni and cheese, grilled cheese. If they came across samples in our local organic market, I still let them indulge in dairy products, but I didn't bring any of it home. I showed them a video clip demonstrating what ingredients are really contained in a typical ice cream sundae. This made my kids aware of the chemicals and animal by-products—such as feathers and beetle shells—that are commonly contained in processed foods. After watching this, they no longer wanted to eat frozen pizzas, cookies, or candy. During this time, Dave and I watched the movie *Forks Over Knives*. After that, we viewed the film with our kids to reinforce our decision to live plant-based."

Transition Gradually

"All was well for a while," Sharon continued, "until I decided to read the ingredients label on the nondairy cheese I was using—not very healthy, either. I became convinced that my entire family needed to move more toward eating whole foods and avoiding processed products. I gradually stopped buying processed products and went about creating my own healthy substitutes. Cashews blended with nutritional yeast added the creamy texture and cheesy taste to a number of dishes. Gradually, after explaining to them that the processed stuff wasn't healthy and we weren't going to buy it anymore, the kids stopped asking for it. Plus, they loved my new creations! I made sure to make a lot of their favorite dishes, but healthier versions of them, including burritos with black beans, salsa, avocado, and cilantro; lentils with rice; and whole grain pasta with homemade sauce and lots of veggies.

"I encouraged the kids and Dave to help with meal planning and preparation, from choosing recipes and selecting ingredients for dishes and desserts, to washing, peeling, and stirring whatever is cooking. I introduced some new seasonings, and allowed everyone to flavor his or her own meal. We invested in some kitchen equipment for preparation of quick, easy, and delicious dishes—a blender, pressure cooker, food processor, and juicer, and a huge salad bowl."

Give Them Healthy Treats

"I experimented and surprised the kids with healthy treats like black bean brownies, as well as creamy frozen fruit sorbets, chocolate cherry ice cream, cookies, fruit-date-nut pies with cashew cream, and cheesy kale chips made with red pepper, garlic, nutritional yeast, lemon juice, and cannellini beans," Sharon explains. "They were often so excited to get to dessert that they ate the main course without hesitation."

Keep Offering, Even If They Initially Refuse to Try

Sharon recalls, "I made sure that the kids understood why we were changing our diet, and I told them if they tried new things I would also make new treats. Before long, my son, who had always had a strong dislike for chickpeas, tomatoes, and avocados, began to ask for them. Now, they are all among his favorite foods. The first time I made Brussels sprouts roasted in tahini and balsamic vinegar, the kids all loved them and asked for seconds! I had them help me pick out recipes that they thought sounded good, encouraged them to help me in the kitchen, and allowed them to make choices when it came to flavoring certain dishes. Allowing them to have some role in deciding what they wanted to eat—within my guidelines, some flexibility, and a hand in the preparation—was critical in getting them to the table, and to enjoy the experience of eating food that was truly good for them."

Set a Great Example

"Dave quickly got on board once he saw how passionate I was becoming about cooking, and about making certain the kids ate healthfully," Sharon added. "We both knew that we were their role models—that watching us eat this way consistently would inspire them. We continued to express our excitement over finding new recipes that were a hit, and when the kids saw how much we were enjoying them, they had no hesitation in tasting them, too."

Help Them Navigate Social Situations Gracefully

"Social situations were a bit of a challenge at first," Sharon recalls, "but we gradually made our way to a very comfortable place. We explained to the kids that most people—including most of their friends—were eating the Standard American Diet, and that the way we eat may seem a bit 'extreme' to them. I have enjoyed having my kids' friends over for play dates and feeding them green smoothies, black bean brownies, healthy nachos, hummus burritos, and frozen banana berry 'ice cream' . . . and then telling their parents when they came to pick them up that their child ate black beans, kale, and chickpeas. On occasion I save some for the parents to try—almost every time, it's been a huge hit and they asked for the recipe. For my kids, having their friends enjoy the same dishes reinforced that healthy food can taste great to everyone.

"I also have made plant-exclusive meals when relatives were over for holidays; these have been well received, even by the other kids in the family, which also made my kids feel great. When the kids are invited to a friend's house to play, I call the parents in advance and explain the way that we eat and tell them I will send a snack to share. No one has ever acted offended and we often receive compliments on the treats. If they go to a party, I explain to the hosts in advance and if they don't offer to make accommodations—which they almost always do—I feed the kids ahead of time. I encourage them to explain that they choose to eat this way—because they do—not that they 'can't have' certain things. They enjoy sharing their kale chips with friends in the cafeteria, and when other kids see them, they ask what they are—and they almost always like them! When we go to restaurants, we call ahead or look up the menu online to find suitable options, and usually come prepared with a small bag of condiments with which to flavor our choices."

Expose Your Lifestyle to Like-Minded People

Sharon continues: "An important aspect of choosing a lifestyle that is different from the norm is to have social support. The same goes for kids. I make certain to bring them to vegan potlucks, festivals, parties, and events. They have learned that there are many other people, including kids, who make the decision to eat the way we do. They have watched a number of movies and documentaries on healthy food, and have seen several plant-based doctors speak. Although a lot of it may have been over their heads, they understand the basic concept that what they eat now has a tremendous role in determining their health later in life. I also made certain to expose them to other issues related to our food choices, such as the impact on the environment and the animals. That way, in case there is peer pressure down the road, they will have a number of reasons for wanting to stay on a healthy path. They have really enjoyed meeting other kids who eat as they do, and have discovered that some of their teachers and a few classmates eat plant-based, too. It's important to them to know that they are not alone."

Don't Give In: Be Confident in Knowing You Are Doing the Right Thing for Your Kids

"There may come a time when you feel unsure that you are doing the right thing—such as when all of the other kids are chowing down on Halloween candy—and you have sent your child in with special healthy treats," Sharon says. "If you have given your kids a good explanation of why it's so important to eat healthy food, they will get over any discomfort quickly. Kids need to know that you are confident in what you are doing—and that it is to protect them because you love them. You may feel from time to time as though you're burned out; I will be the first to admit that there are days that I wish I could just pull up at a drive-thru and pick up a healthy dinner, instead of having to cook. But I think about how much I love my kids, and then a little time in the kitchen doesn't seem so bad."

Always Be Prepared

Says Sharon: "I always make sure that we have some type of bean dip, nut butters, and plenty of fruits and vegetables in the fridge. We never travel anywhere without snacks—fresh or dried fruits, hummus and sprouted grain bread, carrot and celery sticks—so we are never caught hungry without plant-based, unprocessed options. To save time during the week, on the weekends I often prepare beans and grains in big batches for the week. Together with keeping the fridge well stocked with lots of veggies, this means I can throw together a meal pretty quickly. I rely on what I like to call 'the five S's' for plant-based meals: soups, salads, smoothies, sandwiches, and sautés. We have a large salad daily—easy to create quickly using the food processor. I make delicious dressings in the blender, along with bean dips and nut butters for sandwiches and snacks. I also make up a big batch of bean vegetable soup, easy to do quickly using the pressure cooker. I vary the flavors by trying new beans, grains, vegetables, spices, nuts, and seeds, keeping it interesting for all of us. We have a lot of fun coming up with creative desserts, like ice creams, chocolate mousse made with avocado, puddings made with chia seeds, fruit pies, and truffles made with dried fruits, nuts, seeds, and cocoa powder.

"All in all, this has been a very positive transition for all of us. I now feel much more in control of our health destiny. We rarely get sick anymore, even with colds, and when we do, it's very brief and mild. We all have lots of energy and passion for sharing our experience and inspiring others to take control of their health. My kids tell me that they don't feel uncomfortable about eating differently than other people; in fact, they are proud that the way we eat is best for our health, for the animals, and for the planet. I'm so proud of them and the way they have adapted. I hope that this inspires others to consider transitioning their family to a plant-based diet."

Let's Hear from the McRae Kids Themselves

Twins Tess and Marcie, and younger brother Evan McRae—sixteen and twelve, respectively—have now been eating plant-based for over six years. I asked them to tell their story about the family decision to go plant-based—what was hard for them, what was easy, and what their suggestions are for other families.

"When the three of us heard from our parents that we were no longer eating dairy products, we burst into tears!" explained Tess. "I felt confused and lost. I had grown up eating these things and I was in denial that they were being taken away from me." Evan recalls being "quite awestruck and depressed. Even before I actually started eating more greens, I felt deprived." Marcie remembers feeling "upset, angry, and frustrated." She says, "The three of us each dealt with the changes in the same way. Our change to completely plant-based eating was very gradual. Although we were immediately no longer served dairy products at home, we gradually stopped sampling them in grocery stores. We also started to eat plant-based processed food substitutes. We ate like this for about a year and a half, gradually eating more fruits and vegetables and less processed foods."

Marcie continues, "For all three of us, the hardest part of going plant-based was and still is how our food choices affect our relationships with friends and family. Some people are not very supportive and are sometimes even skeptical of the decisions we make. Our friends do not really understand why we choose to eat this way. It's also hard when you think that these same friends and family members will probably have health problems from their lifestyles. Yet it's hard trying to get people to eat differently when they don't want to."

The kids go on to explain, "The easiest part is definitely the food! Our taste buds have changed. Before, all three of us were very picky eaters; now we eat and enjoy almost everything we are offered. We enjoy helping make our meals. In the mornings, we usually make oat cereal with fruit, like an apple or an orange. For lunches, we have sandwiches with homemade hummus and greens, and green smoothies with fruits, vegetables, and seeds. Mom or Dad makes the smoothies for us in the morning and we take them to school in bottles. Dinners usually are from recipes Mom finds on the internet, in cookbooks, or she comes up with something on her own. We have a few favorite dishes that we eat about once a week, but otherwise our dinners have a lot of variety. We normally have rice—red and black are our favorites—and/or beans—with dinner. Sometimes we also have a salad with lots of vegetables first. For dinner we usually eat a soup or stir-fry with vegetables and spices. Desserts and sweet treats are usually fruit."

When I asked Tess, Marcie, and Evan their advice for other youths going plant-based, they said, "Most of our classmates and friends are very set in their ways and think that we must feel deprived by our diet. This is not true—by not eating animal products, you are getting healthier with delicious food! If you are already following this diet and are not getting support, we suggest that you hold your head high and continue to make good, healthy choices. In the end, you will be the one who lives a healthy life!" As for their advice to parents, they say, "Making this choice is one of the best things you can do for your kids. You will set a great example. It may seem like it is hard, but the results of making this change are so good for you."

SOCIAL SITUATIONS, FAMILY GATHERINGS, AND FOOD PUSHERS

You may already have been challenged by friends or family who, upon discovering you are making new food choices, blindside you with their lack of support. This can show up in the form of anything from food pusher tactics and critical comments to blatant hostility. And heaven help us when we hit the holidays, and the hallowed family-heirloom recipe Christmas cookies make their annual appearance. The pressure to partake can seem incessant, and you run the risk of being the family outcast should you dare to decline a glass of the annual eggnog. This can come right up against your food choice line in the sand. You might argue that one bite can't hurt. Yet some find that a few bites of standard festive fare launches a sleigh ride into dietary darkness and they can't come up for air until January. A few days of frosted everything and your brown rice will taste like dirt. Taste change is a two-way street.

Response Systems

It's best to be prepared for these dietary challenges. When confronted either directly or subtly, you have a choice. You can allow the confrontation to undermine your resolve, or you can use it as an opportunity to eat for yourself, practice an understanding of human nature, grow self-confidence, exercise compassion for others, be a role model for the plant-based lifestyle, and be a resource for the inquisitive. It helps to realize that though it may have nothing to do with your intentions, when you start to make choices toward a healthy lifestyle, those around you who are used to your previous patterns of eating may feel threatened. To them, it might feel as if opting for something other than the status quo is a criticism of their lifestyle. Their motivation is probably to keep you anchored in familiar family or friend traditions. Rocking the boat can create discomfort. This is why making such comments as "I'm eating healthier now!" can elicit defenses from friends and family. It's as if by saying you are eating healthier, you are pointing an accusing finger at their bad habits—even though you said nothing of the kind. And not one of us likes that.

When we see it from this perspective, it can give us new insights into how to talk about our choices. This is where some understanding, prepared response systems, and a little bit of practice will help. Demonstrating to those you care about that you still value them—and that you don't feel you are superior to them because of how you eat—is your best ally. The discomfort we detect in ourselves in reaction to negative comments, or simply lack of support, are all offshoots of the same issue: It hooks our latent, lurking limbic fear of being cut off from the clan. Perhaps a mismatch for our modern world, this fear is probably a carryover from our ancient urge to be accepted by the group, ensuring survival. Viewing the situation from this perspective can help. Making as little fuss as possible about your new approach to eating—as excited about it as you may be—is usually the best strategy, especially as you are just getting started. This can be tough, as you may be eager to share the good news about what you are learning about plant-based living with your loved ones and friends. Plus, it seems the minute you start eating healthier, everyone around you becomes a nutritionist. In one way or another, they seem to want to rescue you from dietary deficiency. Overlooking their own health and weight problems, they are suddenly urgently concerned with how much protein you are getting. Try to understand where this might be coming from—most likely they are feeling your change as a departure from them, or it is a reminder of their own dietary shortcomings.

In the same fashion, it's best not to sit down to Thanksgiving dinner and announce to everyone, "I don't eat anything with a mother or a face!" Even though it may be true, to make such an announcement is to inspire naysayers to jockey for position to wait and watch for you to fall short. Human nature being what it is, it simply invites defensive posturing, cloaked in offense and attacks. There are better ways to go about sending the message, and maintaining family harmony, that will be more effective in sowing seeds of interest and inquiry. Going about your own plant-based business, sharing great-tasting food, and underplaying the attention on *you* can have an entirely different, more positive effect than making broad announcements and preaching at the supper table. Sometimes a quick way of deflecting attention from yourself is best.

Three Strategies for Handling Persistent Food Pushers

There's more than one way to say no. As you gain more confidence, you will become increasingly comfortable with "No, thank you," "I've had enough," and "I'm going to pass." But it doesn't hurt to have an arsenal of strategies at the ready. The following have all worked like a charm for me—simply add your own spin. Rehearsing responses and role-playing upcoming scenarios in advance can help, too. With a little creativity and practice you'll come up with your own ideas to add to the list.

The booked solid strategy: To the arm-twisting "Don't you want some cheesecake? It's Mom's original recipe!" I'll pat my belly and say, "I'm booked! I couldn't eat another bite!" Immediately follow this with a comment to take the attention off of you and onto something else—such as the hostess—in an absolutely sincere way, such as, "The centerpiece flowers are so gorgeous, Aunt Jo—are they from your garden?" Of my three strategies, this is the one I've used most often. With a little practice it will become easy.

READER TIP: FOOD PUSHERS

"Your 'how to handle food pushers' strategies helped me a lot this Thanksgiving! I was better prepared for situations that arose. One situation in particular comes to mind.

"As all fifteen guests finished serving themselves buffet style, and sat down at the table, the hostess—also the cook—stood behind me and said, 'So, this is how a vegetarian eats!'

"It drew everyone's attention toward me, just as everyone was starting to eat—the majority eating turkey. No, I didn't launch into a ten-minute explanation of plant-based diets. I simply said, 'Everything looks great, Cathy! I especially like your Brussels sprouts.' She sat down to eat and everyone went about his or her business. Disaster averted and the meal went very well."

—P. David Rij, San Diego

The eat-it-later strategy: To someone trying to get you to take a slice of pecan pie: "Oh, that looks so good! Could I please take some and have it later?"

The push-it-around strategy: To insistent entreaties to try the [fill in the blank], take a small helping anyway, and simply push it around on your plate. At first you might feel a little uncomfortable not eating the food—especially if you are used to saying yes, or to cleaning your plate.

Honestly? People don't really care what you are eating. Most people are conditioned to encourage you to eat and act like something's wrong with you if you don't. It's really nothing personal at all—simply social conditioning. They may pester you to eat more, to try another bite, to put that pie on your plate—but in seconds the conversation is off to something else. Keep in mind that a lot of food pushing is actually hospitality with calories. People want us to feel welcome and comfortable, and traditionally that means food. We, not wanting to appear rude or ungrateful, feel obliged to accept. Turn the situation around by accepting hospitality in other ways, such as responding to "Would you like some turkey?" with "No, thank you, but I'd love more of that gorgeous salad!"

The plant-based lifestyle, like any other change, is caught more than taught. You will win more hearts by attraction via your own kindness, courtesy, success, and delicious food. Like it or not, we are each ambassadors for change. How we speak and conduct ourselves makes a huge difference. Deportment!

FOOD ADDICTIONS OR ADDICTIVE FOODS?

There's another kind of food pusher that isn't human—and that can be the food itself. If we aren't compelled to eat, then our chances for survival are shot. However, this desire can go awry, and we can feel overwhelmingly urged to feed in the presence of highly palatable foods. The act of eating itself stimulates pleasure centers in the brain. Yet when we eat hyper-flavored, sugary, processed foods—the sweetness of which is no longer buffered by fiber, vitamins, and other constituents of whole foods—that system can become dysfunctional, making these edibles irresistible and urging us to eat more. And not because we need the energy, but because our brain is responding to these substances in much the same way it might respond to addictive drugs. Levels of dopamine, endogenous opiates, and serotonin—our feel-good biochemistry—rise, elevating mood while blunting the signals that tell us we've had enough and making it easy to overeat. Over time, your system can adapt to the stimulation, fanning the flames of desire for these foods.

But does an "addictive" response to certain foods an addict make? The research is still in its infancy, and to label yourself as such might be helpful, or it might be counterproductive. Popular references to the terms *addiction* and *disorder*, when it comes to food and eating, can be confusing, making it hard to tease the terms apart for an accurate perspective. Some individuals are more sensitive to this effect of hyper-palatable food than others—you'll find listings in the Resource section so you can investigate further. Yet calling this food addiction and disease is both a scientific and a societal question that continues to be investigated.[6,7]

The issues here are complex, and I don't presume to know all the answers. What I do know is that I used to consider myself hopelessly addicted to sweets. For me, this situation has been transformed with the very tools presented in this book, a synergy of plant-based eating, physical activity, and cultivating some mastery over thinking patterns. Because of this, I'm reluctant to cheer on "I'm a food addict" claims without considering other factors.

Undereating Drives Overeating

Understanding the origins of the urge to eat—and overeat—hyper-caloric edibles, in spite of our better judgment, designs to do otherwise, and straining waistbands, is pivotal to understanding and mastering the challenges these foods present. Before any conversation about food addictions can begin, let's expose the single biggest reason we find ourselves helpless at the edge of the bowl of cookie dough. Hunger left unsatisfied day after day—frequently the fate of the career dieter and those aspiring to lose weight by chronically "cutting back"—builds a mountain of deprivation that routinely collapses in a desperate demise we all recognize: out-of-control eating, usually of everything least compatible with our weight loss goals. Once this problem has been addressed by satisfying our hunger through eating abundantly of whole plant foods, we can take an honest look at the addictive properties of certain foodstuffs.

Hooking the Survival Instinct

We are, along with many critters in the animal kingdom, opportunistic eaters by nature. Hardwired for survival, we are by instinct drawn like a magnet to the richest, most energy-dense foods because, historically, they increased our chances of getting enough fuel to stick around. Our earliest human ancestors had their daily work cut out for them: search for, procure, and consume whatever edibles they could find or forage. Energy-dense foods were an obvious draw because they offered a rich energy source relative to effort expended. This instinctive prizing and consumption of high-calorie fare improved our odds of survival—a taste hierarchy that pulled us to pound down the calories whenever the opportunity might present itself. That pull is still very much alive in our bodies today. It doesn't matter to our limbic instincts that these days we can simply store calories for tomorrow in our pantries and refrigerators instead of carrying them around on our bellies and thighs.

The uber-rich pastries and high-fat meats presented to us modern humans—sometimes multiple times a day—would blow our ancestors' unibrow hair back. They have that same effect on our attention and appetites today as they always have, inviting us to consume more as a hedge against tomorrow's famine or long, deprived winter, which for most of us never comes. Abundant and easy to access in our modern food supply, these foods hand over a reward of immense dietary energy with very little effort on our part. In light of our ancestry, they provide our bodies with a veritable survival jackpot.

> **EAT! MORE! NOW!**
> When foods are highly refined—recall the processed continuum—more of their surface area is exposed to your tongue, making their taste even more pronounced. Your brain fires off urgent signals to "Eat! More! Now!" This may have worked well for our ancestors, when periods of food abundance were peppered with periods of famine. But these days, it just makes it too easy for us to get fat.

Sugar and Fat: From Sweet Seasoning to Habit Forming?

Inextricably bound with our survival instinct is the drive to enjoy the pleasurable biochemical cascade produced in response to eating high-sugar, high-fat foods such as sweets and chocolate.[8] This sweet reward explains why many people can have difficulty controlling the consumption of foods high in sugar when continuously exposed to them.[9] Chronic sugar consumption, and the altered brain chemistry that can result, has been found to be habit-forming in some people. As they experience dopamine depletion and sugar withdrawals, they can experience cravings. This explains some of the difficulty you might experience when letting go of highly refined foods.

Unfortunately, the food industry exploits these cravings. Added sugar is everywhere—usually accompanied by fat—and used in approximately 75 percent of packaged foods purchased in the United States.[10] These foods are laboratory modified to hammer the dopamine pleasure cascade, pushing us to pound down more and more unhealthy foods. This is why you may find that even *thinking* about the foods that create this feel-good cycle for you get your feet moving in the direction of the candy stash before you are even aware. And with the promise of the dopamine rush, it's no mystery why stress can drive us straight to the cookie jar.

Overeating inspired by overstimulating edibles is simply a biological challenge, not a character flaw.[11] The key to curbing cravings is to first address their basic cause by simply eating enough whole plant foods. Remember, the rules of satiety function optimally in a whole food, plant-based environment. You can't count on whole foods to keep you trim when also consuming apple fritters and triple macchiatos. Studies show that when rats are fed healthy chow, based on their natural foods, they easily maintain their ideal weight simply by relying on their hunger and fullness cues. But given the chance to eat chocolate as desired, their energy intake increases by 84 percent. Within 120 days, their weight can balloon by 49 percent.[12] Sounds like the rat equivalent of our holiday season.

Does this mean you have to stick to the human equivalent of rat chow and never eat chocolate again? No, but it does mean that you'll need to avoid going hungry for days on end, and responsibly manage your food environment. The teaspoon of brown sugar you might put on your morning oatmeal isn't the problem. But it's wise to limit intake, become aware of hidden sources to avoid the aftereffects, and respect your own sugar sensitivity. It's also another good reason to avoid packaged, processed foods. Learn to harness some mental muscle—more in chapter 13 (page 174)—in the presence of compelling edibles by cultivating a practice that trains you in the skills of reaction intervention. That way, when faced with the siren call of these foods, increasingly you will be able to not only moderate your eating but also pause and ask yourself: Does real food sound good? If whole food doesn't appeal at that moment, then perhaps it is the voice of your instinctive drive for energy-dense anything that you are hearing, and not necessarily real hunger. Or perhaps you are simply in the midst of a hedonic moment. Nothing wrong with that, yet strung together in rapid succession such interludes will be problematic for your progress. Discriminatory muscle can be built with practice.

People differ in their carrying capacity for foods that overstimulate their appetites. Some are able to enjoy them intermittently; others are more sensitive to their pull. Once the guilt is gone, we gain rational perspective and can take specific steps to get this more-calories-per-minute monkey off our backs. It gives you some leverage for solving the problem. Think carefully about what you keep in the kitchen. It may be in your best interests to, for now, eliminate from your immediate environment any foods that have rendered you helpless in the past. As a result, the insidious itch to indulge will fade. Honesty about what is true for you—paired with building the practice of eating abundantly of whole plant foods to satisfy hunger—is your ticket to personal success.

Whatever your transition strategy, once you've developed a solid collection of "go-to" meals and systemized kitchen readiness, you've got the components of the plant-based lifestyle in place so that it starts to work *for* you. When you're certain that you know how to surround yourself with delicious and satisfying food, and keep it within reach wherever your day takes you, you are ready to embrace the Ten-Day Plant-Based Makeover in the next chapter with confidence and enthusiasm.

CHAMPION

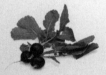

The Road to Mastery

CHAPTER 11

The Ten-Day Plant-Based Makeover

You've now reached the Champion stage of the journey, which, from its name, you might think is the most detailed of them all. Actually, you now have all the basics you need. The qualities of the Champion are grounded in practice. Practice is how mastery is obtained, embellished, and refined. It is the traction that carries you forward with continued improvement and minimizes backsliding. Once you see this, you sail onward with a whole new, bright and shining, positive perspective.

The Champion also stays mindful of the fact that the progression through the levels of the journey, rather than being a straight ascending line, is more a spiral, yet with deep roots—like stabilizing, guiding moorings at each curve. The preceding levels continue to provide stability and support. You still wear your Scout hat as you continue to learn more about plant-based living. You retain Rookie status as you keep trying new foods and recipes. You get better and better at taking plant-based eating on the road. Understanding and embracing this brilliant synergy are the hallmarks of the Champion. The Champion adventure—the Ten-Day Plant-Based Makeover option—simply invites you to focus on fine-tuning the skills you've already put into place.

THE TEN-DAY PLANT-BASED MAKEOVER

The Ten-Day Plant-Based Makeover is simply eating plant-based whole foods for ten continuous days. Using the systems and practices with which you have growing familiarity and expertise, you are now prepared for this. Implement it whenever you are ready. As a matter of fact, it may already be exactly how you are dining every day. The Makeover simply gives you a structured time frame to see how your practices measure up. And if you need guidance for "out of the fire" transition, or have been looking for an excuse or a little push to take you "all the way" for a focused plant-exclusive excursion, here it is.

Why ten days? The cells of your taste buds renew continuously, regenerating about every ten days.[1] Their vulnerability—think of all the times you've burned or frozen your tongue—has made this adaptive, rapid cell turnover necessary. It also means that your taste preferences can be re-created just as quickly—a real plus when building new favorite flavors.

Take as much time as you want to get ready. This way, you will experience full immersion in the whole food, plant-based lifestyle—*yet not before you've practiced*, and become somewhat skilled at, the basics. You may find that your own rhythm of additions and eliminations is suiting your needs to a T. Perfect enough. At the same time, there are some distinct advantages to the Ten-Day Plant-Based Makeover. First, it's the most direct way to experience the multiple benefits of the plant-based lifestyle full on. The recalibration of taste buds alone is going to give your program a decided boost. In just a few days of exclusive whole food, plant-based eating, the flavors of vegetables and whole grains will become more pronounced, increasing the pleasure of eating. Fruits will taste like candy. Weight loss is almost always a side effect. And if you have your baseline blood chemistry numbers checked before you start—such as cholesterol and triglyceride levels—you will be able to see how quickly changes can occur. This will also give you more tools of measurement to affirm your progress. You can do anything for ten days. With the confidence of ten days, you may just find yourself adding on another ten days, then another ten days . . .

Getting Ready

While the Makeover doesn't require any special food direction other than that already provided, it invites you to create a block of time for practicing all the elements in concert.

1. Establish a ten-day period of time that you know is most likely to support your quest. There's no "perfect time," and the longer you delay looking for just such a thing, the less likely you are to find it. While scheduling a time when you are busy is just as good as any other, circling two days before Christmas as your start date is probably not optimal.

2. Stock your refrigerator, pantry, workplace, and every place else you eat with appropriate foods and supplies. Divest them of everything that isn't. This is a statement of intention. It sends the message that you mean business, and is a powerful way to support yourself. Use the food groups guide from chapter 3 (page 28) and the shopping list (page 216) to organize your ten-day project.

Juice for the Journey

The Ten-Day Plant-Based Makeover needn't be limited to your plate. Let it broaden to include the other important elements of a healthy, happy, plant-based lifestyle. That means the food, the fitness, *and* the frame of mind. It will help you move forward. Picture your journey as a cart with two wheels. Whole plant foods comprise the cart. The two wheels carrying it forward are physical activity and mental mastery. What happens when a cart has one wheel smaller than the other? It keeps going in circles. And with just one wheel, well, we don't get far at all.

Give yourself important "juice" for the journey. Regular physical activity—as simple as a daily walk—and centering time and mindfulness practice are pivotal. Perfect timing. These are directly ahead in section six (page 159).

PLANT-BASED TRANSFORMATION: J.C. HUGHES'S JOURNEY

J.C. Hughes found "immersion" style—of which the Ten-Day Plant-Based Makeover is an example—a successful way to launch his plant-based journey. Two years ago, J.C.'s type 2 diabetes was raging out of control, his blood pressure was climbing, and his weight had hit an all-time high of 265. Feeling understandably sluggish and completely out of shape, J.C. became aware of the plant-based Get Healthy Marshall Program and contacted Marshall, Texas, mayor Ed Smith and his wife, Amanda, to find out more about it.

J.C.—the public works and water utilities director for the city of Marshall, Texas—had made moves to improve his health before. Thirty years earlier he had given up a three-pack-a-day smoking habit. Over the years, his weight ballooned and he realized his lifestyle choices were killing him. In his words, "I likened my diet to a slow-based death plan. I needed to try something, but with so many so-called diet plans promoted in the media and online, I wanted something that made sense, sounded healthy, and was easy to follow. Like a lot of folks, I had tried dozens of different diets with limited or short-lived success; what I really needed was a lifestyle change. Having grown up in rural east Texas, our family always had a garden as a kid and my family ate mostly vegetables. A plant-based program was like going back to my roots.

"Prior to converting to plant-based, my normal breakfast consisted of eggs, lots of bacon, hash browns—heavy on the salt—biscuits laden with margarine and jelly, and several cups of sugar with my coffee. Lunch was usually a ham sandwich with mayo, chips, and one or two large Cokes. For supper, chicken every way you can cook it—preferably fried or barbecued—and gravy, milk, and butter on anything. Take-out and fast food was the rule of the day—usually burgers, something fried, or pizza."

When he first started the plant-based program, J.C. experienced a rapid 35-pound weight loss. He continues to lose weight and, working with his doctor, has reduced and dropped several of his medications. "An unexpected benefit is that my overall temperament has leveled off—no ups and downs—and my energy is unreal for someone my age," he adds. "What really worked for me was a twenty-one-day plan. Set a goal to try plant-based for at least twenty-one days, and then compare your results—that gave me all I needed to move forward! I believe this type of plan is easy and the results after just twenty-one days are amazing."

He continues, "At the same time, I admit that for a while I was eating about 98 percent plant-based, as my favorite late-night snack was a 'small' ice cream sandwich. Why? I know what works for me and I have found at this point in my journey that a small reward satisfies my bad cravings; in the long run, it will be a lot easier to drop the few small snacks and then really see the huge rewards of going 100 percent. After about six months, I dropped the snack. It also took me a while to get the butter out of my diet. I gradually stopped eating foods that I normally used butter on and a few weeks after that, I lost the desire for the taste."

"The hardest thing has been giving up meat and sugar," explains J.C. "I had a deep craving for meat at first, but over time—as it was when I quit smoking—the craving slowly left. Sugar was the same way. Time was what it took for me, but I did develop a few tricks: 1) I cleansed the cabinets and fridge of any non-plant-based foods; 2) I placed a lot of fruits in a bowl on the kitchen cabinet as a temptation to grab fruit for a snack; 3) I placed a bowl of fruit and plant-based snacks on a table in the den, where we watch television; 4) I replaced my daily Cokes with water, and set a goal of drinking a 1.5-liter container of water daily, which also fills me up and reduces my cravings; and 5) I totally avoid areas of the grocery store that harbor non-plant-based items! As for restaurants, I have conditioned myself to immediately ask for a vegan or plant-based menu, not even looking at other portions of the menu. I try to frequent locations I know have plant-based menu items."

I asked J.C. whether he has experienced any setbacks along the way. "After the initial major weight loss, I hit a long-term plateau in my weight loss and reduction in meds," he replies. "Everyone I talked to said this is normal and to hang in there. I slowly started to move away from the plant-based plan. When I received my semiannual lab results, I had gained back 10 pounds, my blood pressure and blood sugar were up, and I was not feeling as well. My doctor was tempted to modify my meds, even adding back some we had reduced. That was all the motivation I needed. I got back into plant-based, and the latest doctor's report showed my weight down again. Now I am more motivated than ever—my wife is also supportive and is moving more toward a plant-based lifestyle herself. My next goal is to reach a 100 percent plant-based lifestyle."

J.C. adds, "There's another important benefit of a more personal nature that should be mentioned. When I first started talking to other men following the plant-based lifestyle, they would describe their benefits of permanent weight loss, reversing high blood pressure and diabetes, reduction and elimination of medicines, etc. Yet in every case, just as I was about to walk away, they almost all—using the same exact words and whisper tone, like it was an inside guy secret—added, 'Hey, you will notice you can perform better.' Needless to say, that got my attention! It was almost comical the way they expressed this benefit from their plant-based program, stating it so softly, almost in passing." This benefit is not uncommon and has been reported across the board by multiple physicians advocating a plant-based lifestyle, such as John McDougall, MD, who reports, "The same diet that closes the arteries to the heart (heart attacks) and brain (stroke) also closes [other] arteries . . . Fortunately, with a change in diet and a little exercise most of our patients are able to lower their blood pressure and get off of their ' . . . deflating' medications . . . by reversing the underlying atherosclerosis. My male patients (and sometimes their mates) often share with me tales of their renewed vigor and vitality. Now there's a valid reason to eat vegetables."[2]

Adds J.C., "Yes, I've noticed an ever-improving difference. This is an added benefit to my greatly improving health, and helps keep me in a plant-based frame of mind. Maybe it's time that the possible positive benefits of a plant-based program came out of the back rooms!"

"As I keep telling people," J.C. continues, "a plant-based program is not a diet; it is a lifestyle modification. You will never regret converting to a plant-based lifestyle. You have to develop a deep understanding that you are *not* giving up anything, you are replacing past food choices with plants and fruit, and nothing is lost except weight, medication dependency, and gradually worsening health. More than anything, it gives me a good feeling inside that I have made a full circle back to my plant-based roots with country gardens. If it comes from a garden or off a tree, it has to be good for me and my family!"

THE KEY SUPPORTING PLAYERS

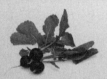

*Exercise and
Mastering Strength of Mind*

CHAPTER 12
Fit for the Cause

THE PROFOUNDLY POSITIVE EFFECT OF PHYSICAL ACTIVITY ON YOUR JOURNEY

Walking away with the award for best performance in the role of supporting player in transition to the plant-based lifestyle is exercise. Though people may think the primary benefits of exercise are burning calories and building muscle, there's a bigger story to tell beyond a stronger heart and a better figure. The more important benefit that physical activity delivers is its effect on your brain and your ability to respond to the demands of change. It has profound effects on cognitive ability, brain function, mood, and mental health. Easily accessible, it does all of this by boosting brainpower and bestowing a good attitude along with a long-term sense of well-being. *This energizes lifestyle transformation.* The food is your first focus on the plant-based journey, but in this chapter you'll find out how physical activity gives your whole project more optimism, energy, and momentum.

MOVING THE BODY BROADENS THE MIND

Exercise has also been found to stimulate neurogenesis—the creation of new brain cells, or neurons. Neurogeneticists are now studying exercise not because they're interested in exercise per se, but because of its potential to build a better brain. Clearly, moving your body helps keep your brain growing.[1]

Movement as Mood Enhancer

Exercise fires up the very same regions of your brain as other mood enhancers, like highly palatable foods and addictive drugs.[2] Both result in a similar cascade of biochemical responses—your internal antidepression mechanism.[3] As soon as you start putting one foot in front of the other, levels of dopamine rise. This sprouts new dopamine receptors in your brain's motivation center, delivering fresh levels of initiative and inspiring neural pathways that build a new healthy habit: exercise.[4] Movement is the natural condition of the body, and engaging in robust physical activity keeps our brains and psyches at peak performance. The fact that physical inactivity contributes to weight gain[5] might not be so much that we aren't burning calories but that we're missing the boost in well-being that we, in a misguided attempt to raise our spirits, seek out in junk food instead of just going for a walk.

Movement as Agent for Positive Change

The lifestyle shifts you are making—changing the way you think about food and eating—demand building new systems and creating new practices. These require the ability to adapt to change. Exercise is the simplest, most direct way to give muscle to the building blocks of your brain, sparking the creation of new synapses and bestowing beneficial effects on memory and executive function.[6] This expedites positive transformation by sparking connections between past experiences and present action, planning and organizing, strategizing, and attention to important details[7]—directly related to making the important shifts necessary on this journey.

Exercise enhances the expression of a protein in your brain called brain-derived neurotrophic factor, or BDNF. BDNF plays an important role in mood regulation, brain cell growth, and learning. Without BDNF, our brains aren't able to take in new information or make new cells. These are the biochemical basics for learning something new, such as those demanded by making lifestyle changes. The exercise-induced rush of hormones to your brain mixes with BDNF, nourishing neurons—somewhat like scattering fertilizer on your flower garden. It's like "Miracle-Gro for the brain," says John J. Ratey, MD, associate clinical professor of psychiatry at Harvard Medical School. The fact that BDNF has such a strong impact on neuron growth is profoundly good news. "What it means is that you have the power to change your brain. All you have to do is lace up your running shoes."[8]

BDNF also plays this important role in brain cell growth and learning by enhancing what is known as brain *neuroplasticity*. Neuroplasticity is the biological process by which your brain responds to its environment. This makes it possible for you to form new connections and learn new behaviors necessary to carry on. Neuroplasticity is what allows you to file away new experiences, store new knowledge, and adapt to change. This ability to change our mental models—patterns of thinking—lets us open the door to transformative learning. The result is the acquisition of new skills that you need.[9] Without neuroplasticity, you remain cemented in old habits, perspectives, and ways of thinking about things, making neuroplasticity a clearly desirable commodity when implementing lifestyle shifts. Inertia of body leads to inertia of mind.

By stimulating the BDNF growth factor, you become mentally poised to create new systems of practice that support your improved, healthy lifestyle. Think of it as a booster shot for building better habits. And though we still have a lot to learn about how exercise impacts BDNF, the existing evidence tells us that the exercise-induced up-regulation of BDNF expression plays a role in both enhancing cognitive function and upgrading your mood.

MOVE YOUR LEGS TO DEFOG YOUR BRAIN

Your calf muscles are your peripheral pump, and their contraction causes a surge in circulation. When sitting or reclining, the calves check out of the program. Is it any wonder that after sitting for a period of time you start to nod off? Standing and moving about gets the calves back in gear, stimulating the lymph system—your detox agent—and squeezing blood out of the lower extremities and back to your heart for oxygen. This replenishes the brain supply, restoring mental alertness.

Now that you know that exercise builds brain as well as brawn, how do you get started, or simply optimize what you are currently doing? Perhaps you're already getting regular physical activity. But if you haven't gotten off the couch since the Clinton administration, it's time to get moving. Let's start by seeing whether you're sitting too much and take it from there.

ARE YOU SITTING TOO MUCH?

Another way to look at physical activity and the brain is by examining the damaging effects left in the wake of *lack* of exercise. It is not uncommon for people to spend most of their waking day sitting at computers, in cars, on couches, and in restaurants, with relatively idle muscles. Just the process of moving about to procure food required our ancestors to take far more steps each day than we do now. We've become more efficient at extracting energy from the environment, keeping us well fed, but now less energy output is required for us to subsist. Our inherent requirement for healthy movement and the activity demands of our modern lifestyle are at an all-time mismatch. This has added to the explosion of health concerns from high levels of inactivity.[10]

We now know that all this time we spend sitting has become a serious health hazard, resulting in what has become known as "inactive physiology" or "sitting disease." It accelerates disease biomarkers such as raised cholesterol and triglycerides, increases incidence of precursors to type 2 diabetes, and has negative effects on your cardiovascular and metabolic systems. Even if you get your workouts in, meeting physical activity guidelines, sitting for prolonged periods can compromise metabolic health.[11] It's called being an active couch potato. The problems of sedentarism extend to brain function. To understand this, all we have to do is look at the positive benefits exercise delivers and note what can happen in its *absence*: the opposite. Reduced neuroplasticity and neurogenesis, increased brain atrophy, and lowered availability and production of neurotransmitters are the result, all of which detract from your ability to effect healthy lifestyle change.

The optimal balance of daily exercise, sedentary time, and non-exercise activity—housework, shopping, puttering, and standing, for example— remains to be exactly detailed. Still, we have enough information about inactive physiology that you should make no delay in adjusting your daily activity patterns to impact the health and well-being of your body and brain in a simple yet fundamental way: by sitting less. Luckily, by structuring breaks for light activity, you will experience immediate benefits. Reversal of disease biomarkers, a better mood, and more clarity of mind are your immediate rewards.

We can be surprisingly unaware of how much time each day, outside of designated exercise and sleep, we spend sitting or reclining. Finding out can be a bit of a shock, but more importantly, a valuable item of discovery.

The Waking Day Metabolic Profile Timeline

The waking day metabolic profile is a tool you can use to help you *become aware* of how much time you spend off your feet. From there, you can set an activity *intention* and *identify* opportunities for sitting less and increasing even non-exercise light activity.[12]

To discover a realistic picture of your sitting versus moving behavior, keep a journal to log your activity levels. Tracking your metabolic profile for a few days will tell you all you need to know. Jot down your activity in thirty-minute blocks during the day for a five-day period. From this activity log, you will be able to *identify* exactly where to start making improvement. Then you can make the micro changes necessary and *practice* incorporating more activity into your day.

Sample Metabolic Profile

This simple example will help you create a metabolic profile of your own:[13]

1. **Awake at 7 A.M. and exercise (60 minutes)**
2. **Prepare and eat breakfast (standing/sitting 45 minutes)**
3. **Drive to work (sitting 45 minutes)**
4. **Work seated at computer workstation (sitting 4 hours)**
5. **Take a lunch break (sitting 60 minutes)**
6. **Work seated at computer workstation (sitting 4 hours)**
7. **Drive home (sitting 45 minutes)**
8. **Prepare and eat dinner (standing/sitting 60 minutes)**
9. **Watch TV and read in seated position (sitting 2.5 hours)**

In this case study example, there are two four-hour blocks of seated behavior at work each day as well as two and a half hours each night of sitting while watching TV and reading. Another ninety minutes are spent seated in the car commuting. Meals were taken sitting down, with light activity for food prep. Add in another eight hours reclining for sleep and this person demonstrates sedentary behavior for nearly twenty-two hours of the day—a staggering 90 percent of his waking time. These time blocks of inactivity are just begging for some activity interventions. It's easy to start making a difference.

The goal of a metabolic profile is to inspire you to add more movement by breaking up and reducing sedentary periods of time during your waking day. Attempt to punctuate these periods with some type of activity every thirty to forty-five minutes. If you lead a sedentary weekend lifestyle, reduce sitting accordingly.

Four Steps to Becoming a More Active Person

You may be very fit, already living an active lifestyle. Or you may be a seden-tarist. The same steps used to plantify your plate can be used to activate your body, or build new levels of fitness.

1. **Become aware. How much activity—or lack of—is showing up in your day? The metabolic profile gives you a tool of discovery.**
2. **Set your intentions. Specify your fitness and physical activity aspirations. For example, do you want to work up to walking for forty-five minutes every day? Run a 5K? Or simply sit less? By how much? Be specific.**
3. **Identify micro changes and dates. Pinpoint the small changes that will be necessary for you to get from where you are to where you want to be. Establish specific dates and times for implementation.**
4. **Practice!**

Case Study: Nichole

Nichole is a perfect example of how this simple system can result in big change. When we started working together, one of Nichole's primary goals—she was already *aware* that exercise had taken a backseat—was to get more exercise. A busy mother of three children under the age of nine, she had a clear *intention*: to build more strength and resiliency. The challenge was to *identify* the small changes she could start to make to become more active and fit, and to spot where in her busy day she could sneak in activity.

Readiness is huge when it comes to doing exercise. And for busy moms, if you have to change your clothes to exercise, that can often seem like too great an obstacle. Since Nichole walks her children to school, she *identified* this as a time to add more activity. She decided to put on her yoga pants first thing in the morning—an important *micro change*—to make slipping in more exercise easier. The effect of this *practice* was immediate. Over the next two weeks, three times each week she was walking extra distances after dropping off the kids. She had become inspired to move more by wearing attire that, to her, suggested movement—yoga pants. From there, she made more micro changes: She started scheduling five-minute targeted workouts into her day, one exercise, one day at a time. And so can you. Sneaking in exercise this way is a very effective, proven strategy for building a more active—and less sedentary—lifestyle.

Small segments of exercise add up, and this approach may be just what you need. Research tells us that short bouts of exercise are just as effective as longer segments for building fitness.[14] Connect regular tasks with physical activity: Perform wall squats while brushing your teeth; complete calf raises while heating up your hot drink for breakfast; practice push-ups against the office wall just before your midmorning break. As physical activity restores brainpower and physical confidence, you will start to notice the brain-building and mood-elevating effects of these fitness breaks, encouraging you to do more as your brain circuitry sends in reinforcements.

Movement Intervention Strategies

Adopting new health-building physical activity means you will need to think outside your usual movement patterns to establish new ones. Simply incorporating more breaks during sedentary time helps—independent of total sedentary time and moderate- to vigorous-intensity activity time—resulting in enhanced mood and reduced waist circumference, body mass index, and triglycerides.[15]

Here are some simple ways to break up those sustained sitting periods at work and home:

- **Stand up and move every time you need to get some water; if you bring your own, take it on a walk while you sip.**
- **Take phone calls standing up.**
- **Rather than email office colleagues, walk to their desks to communicate with them.**
- **Create a standing workstation.**
- **Wear a pedometer to encourage taking steps.**
- **Set a timer on your home computer or phone to alert you to get up every thirty to forty minutes and break up sitting with short bursts of activity, like dashing to the mailbox.**
- **At conferences and meetings, take your seating at the side or back of the room so that you can pepper periods of sitting with stints of standing. For example, sit for forty minutes, stand for twenty.**
- **Take three to five minutes to complete simple yet challenging exercises that require no special equipment. The five-minute workouts provided in *Fit Quickies: 5-Minute Targeted Body-Shaping Workouts* are a perfect example. Short bursts of activity add up, and you can structure it so that by day's end, five minutes at a time, you've completed a full workout.**

Each of these interventions immediately accomplishes two things: 1) restores mental clarity and builds brain function through the brain-enhancing properties of exercise, and 2) offsets the disease-promotion problems related to inactive physiology by breaking up periods of sitting with standing or light activity.

You can also employ specific strategies to help you become more active. This can be as simple as setting out your walking clothes and shoes every evening so that the next day—perhaps when you are least motivated to organize yourself for exercise—you have conveniently made everything ready to go. This can be a complete game changer for incorporating more physical activity—just like having food in the fridge ready to eat makes meals easier.

WHICH EXERCISE AND HOW MUCH?

In addition to sitting less by integrating standing and more non-exercise activity, you'll need designated exercise time that provides a greater challenge, not only for physical fitness but also for the mental vitality so important to healthy lifestyle change. The study of physical inactivity highlights the potential role that all aspects of moving your body can play in impacting your health. In *Fit Quickies* I provide an exercise prescription to clarify what the research tells us about how much of each kind of exercise—cardiorespiratory, strength training, flexibility training, and neuromotor training—we need.[16] The important takeaway is that we need multiple forms of physical challenge to be at our best. Be sure to include each form of challenge two or three times each week for optimal function of both your body and your brain.

> **THE EXERCISE-CONFIDENCE CONNECTION**
> Exercise leads to improvements in emotional outlook and self-esteem, no matter what your size. When people become more active, they also feel more in control of their dietary habits. It also displaces sedentary habits that can lead to snacking, making you more apt to stay on a healthy eating plan.[17]

The exception is cardio, some form of which is recommended several times a week. Much of the research conducted on cognitive enhancement, mood boosting, and increased well-being in relation to physical activity has been done in connection with cardiovascular exercise, defined as continuous, rhythmic movement of the large muscle groups of the body. During cardiovascular activity, your heart rate climbs, your breathing picks up, and you break out in a light sweat. While all that is getting under way, here's how the brain is getting the benefit of your brisk walk or run: extra blood circulates to the brain, bathing your brain cells in oxygen and glucose—which they need to function—and triggering the cascade of brain-building events. As a matter of fact, the more they get, the better they perform. Subjects performing just fifteen minutes of pedaling exercise experienced a significant increase in oxygenated blood to the prefrontal cortex—aka the command center—of the brain, along with a marked increase in alpha brain wave activity.[18] Think of it as your brain on cardio.

Current physical activity guidelines focus on achieving thirty minutes per day—or 150 minutes per week—of moderate to vigorous physical activity. This chunk of time represents only about 3 percent of the time we spend awake. Think of this as the bare minimum. Build up to forty-five minutes to an hour; if you break this up into ten-minute segments as needed, you'll still get the benefit.[19] Aim for every day, and then if you can only hit six days out of seven, consider it a win. If you're nowhere near that amount of activity now, simply start with sitting less and walking more, and work your way up.

This cardiovascular activity can be of varying intensity, and includes everything from a refreshing walk to jogging, running, swimming, biking, or some combination of them all. Mixing in occasional higher intensity activity has been shown to deliver extra goods when it comes to building brainpower and positive mental attitude. Our bodies need to be challenged to keep our brains at peak performance.

While writing this book, I hit the trail every morning for a three-mile run. Sometimes my runs were slower, sometimes faster, sometimes a combination. Not only has it been a good system for baseline fitness, but also it never fails to deliver from the brain-boosting perspective, helping me to creatively connect the dots and mentally integrate related ideas. Each morning upon landing back on the front porch after a run, I'd ask my husband not to talk to me for another twenty minutes so I could dash right to my office, where I would download the inspiration and turns of phrase inspired by the morning ramble through the woods. At first I tried taking a notebook with me, jotting down ideas as they were generated. But I found that stopping to write interrupted the flow and I was better off just retrieving ideas once I got back to my author's nest. You, too, may have experienced firsthand the way brisk activity brings mental clarity and builds new brain connections. Nothing sparks creativity like exercise.

EXERCISING MAKES LOW-CALORIE FOODS MORE APPETIZING

Have you ever noticed that after you exercise, the appeal of healthy food is enhanced? Research backs up this experience. As detected via magnetic resonance imaging (MRI), exercise has been shown to *increase* neural activity in reward-related regions of the brain in response to images of low-calorie foods, while *suppressing* the activation of same when viewing images of high-calorie foods.[20]

Resistance Training

While research tells us that resistance training—also known as strength training—is crucial for building muscle and protecting the joints, which has enormous implications for quality of life, research on the effects of resistance training on learning is still in its infancy. As noted by John Ratey, MD, of Harvard Medical School, "It's difficult to get [lab] rats to pump iron or do yoga."[21] The bulk of brain research connected with resistance training has focused on mood and anxiety, with evidence of improved executive control at the command center of the brain, enhanced memory, and better self-esteem.[22] Additional favorable psychological changes in strength-trained subjects are improvements in perceived confidence in physical capability.[23] These betterments in psychological well-being are essential for making healthy lifestyle choices.

Obstacles to Exercise

With the benefits of exercise so clear, why isn't everyone doing it? Why do so many people drop out once they get started? And why do so many people never get started in the first place? What can you do to ensure that you are one of the "doers," reaping all the rewards that directly advance your plant-based adventure by building new systems, patterns, and habits?

Although understanding the benefits of exercise may be enough to get you started, what keeps you going—in addition to experiencing the benefits of physical challenge—is how you view yourself based on past experiences and current reality when it comes to being physically active. The primary psychological factor to help you stick to an exercise plan is what is known as *self-efficacy*—your confidence in your ability to exercise and be consistent with your workouts. In other words, *thinking* you can successfully do exercise is the most powerful indicator in your ability to stick with it. If you have a long history of failed attempts at exercise, or you have no experience at launching an exercise program, this gives you important information about obstacles that may be getting in your way. In contrast, the more you think you can successfully do exercise, the more likely you are to get moving and stay with it. This is the best argument for starting with whatever level of activity you are confident you will be able to complete.[24]

FROM ZERO TO WALKING

"I weigh over 300 pounds and it hurts to exercise. I sit all day. Is there any hope for me losing this weight?" Sondra asked over the phone.

I restored Sondra's hope by clarifying for her that weight loss is, first, a function of improving her food plan. The Plant-Based Plate is the first stop on the road to getting well. Then, reminding her of the power of physical activity to boost interest in making healthier choices, I asked her whether she was able to stand up. To which she replied, "Yes!"

Sondra was already *aware* that her activity level was virtually zero. Her *intention*, at this point, was to be simply less sedentary. We clarified this to something more specific: a *micro change* of incorporating short periods of *not* sitting or reclining. I suggested to Sondra that she start by standing for five minutes the next day—a start date. From there, we added more five-minute standing periods at other points throughout the day, ten-minute stretching periods, and finally incorporated steps. Within a month, Sondra was walking five, then ten, then fifteen, and finally thirty minutes a day. This is how you string together micro changes for macro results. Sondra is now down over 100 pounds. It all started with simply standing up.

There's another important factor in getting started with exercise, and that is having a personal connection with the benefits exercise will bring you. This means simply finding your "why"—that all-important motivational key we've talked about before when it comes to embarking on the plant-based journey. Saying you want to "eat better"—or start an exercise program—to "be healthier" isn't enough. It's too vague. *You need an emotional connection to what healthy means.* Do you want to have more energy for daily demands, such as shopping at the market and carrying your bags with ease? To be able to dash through the airport to catch a flight? Play with your kids or grand-children? Get ready for that 10K? Or is longevity and quality of life important to you, so that you can live fully as long as you are alive? With a brain that functions well, so you can continue to flourish, create, and live independently? Personal connection is imperative in every single venue, from food to fitness. Finally, unrealistic expectations can be an obstacle. Starting to exercise and expecting it to shed that excess 20 pounds in a month is setting yourself up for disappointment.

Antidotes to Exercise Obstacles

The challenges of self-efficacy and expectation are the below-the-surface issues that may show up as any one of many common reasons that people give for dropping out of—or never even starting—an exercise program. These include being self-conscious about appearance, engaging in negative self-talk and poor body image, lacking time or energy, receiving little support for exercise from family or friends, bad weather, or not having a place to work out.[25] Yet each of these obstacles has an antidote. Being aware of what's at their root can help you disarm them. Lack of time? Plan, organize, and prioritize physical activity. Uninspired to move? Find ways to make activity more enjoyable: Play music to energize your steps, get new walking shoes, walk with a friend or your canine companion. Lack of support? If you can't find anyone locally to connect with, endless resources for connecting with others doing the same thing as you—building a healthy, active lifestyle—abound on the internet.

We all want the benefits of being more fit. I guarantee there's not a single person reading this who wouldn't agree with me that when you exercise—whether it's a short walk, playing catch with your canine, or a full-blown workout—you experience an instant surge in well-being. You feel more energized, yet relaxed. Physical confidence and mental outlook get a decided boost. You simply feel healthier. In other words, health means more than the numbers on a chart. It means having the vitality to do all the things you want to do in life. It means feeling good in your body. It means having a physical resiliency that invites you to be active, rather than the absence of vitality, which holds you back from fully participating in the life that you want.

Once you get your "why" going, this can be enough to get you started with simply walking. Focus on the enjoyment of the walk itself, and don't worry about increasing intensity or time. At first you can start with ten minutes. Make that your intention, and when you've done that every day for a week, you will build self-confidence—just as you have by making simple recipes from templates, or eating lots of whole foods every day. You just raised your self-efficacy factor. That's how you advance success. Literally—when it comes to exercise—one step at a time.

With its profound effect on your brain chemistry, exercise raises your readiness for positive change. It opens the door to possibility and inspires action. It gets your mind ready. Getting excited and energized to get healthier and eat better boosts the journey. Yet how do you harness the mind to help you keep putting one foot in front of the other when it comes to changing your old patterns of eating? In the next chapter, you'll assemble some practical tools for building strength of mind so that you can bridle that inner healthy initiative.

PLANT-BASED TRANSFORMATION: DEBBY'S JOURNEY

"How did I let my weight get so out of control? That is the first thing that comes to my mind when I look back at pictures of me at my heaviest," says Debby. "It wasn't that I did not know how to eat properly and exercise. In the past I had followed a plant-based diet, and been very successful. What had always been missing for me was in the 'mind-set' category. I was never willing to put myself first on the list. My children, husband, job—anything and everything came before taking care of myself. Years of not showing the same consideration for myself as I did for others was affecting more than my weight. The result was a woman who was morbidly obese.

"I love the word *awakening*—what a wonderful way to describe my plant-based journey. Though not a stranger to this wonderful way of eating, I had definitely fallen off the path. About five years ago—due to a family member's crisis, and then a forced career change—I stopped focusing on my own health needs. My food choices had become a reflection of my crazy, stress-filled life. Fast-food and restaurant meals full of fat, sugar, and salt dominated my menu. Stress causes me to eat compulsively, and these types of foods encouraged it. Then, in March 2013, I was 'awakened' by a health crisis.

"Skyrocketing high blood pressure caused a retinal vein occlusion, and bleeding in my left eye. Suddenly my vision was severely compromised. I was told that the 'best' that I could hope for was that my vision would not deteriorate further, but that the condition could lead to blindness. I was immediately placed on two types of blood pressure medication and scheduled for a follow-up visit with the ophthalmologist, at which time he said he would probably be recommending a surgical procedure for my eye. My feelings at the time included fear (I did not want to lose my sight) and anger (at myself because I knew that my eating and lifestyle choices had brought me to this horrible place). Unfortunately, it took the crisis with my eye to wake me up. Even though I knew how to eat a whole food, plant-based diet, I turned to Lani for the extra support that I felt would really benefit me in moving forward in this journey. I also read some of the great plant-based doctors' works, which convinced me that this is the healthiest way of eating for me.

"I am now 90 percent or more whole food, plant-exclusive, with occasional processed treats. I have experienced so many benefits! I have regained my health. My blood pressure—with no medication—is 110/70. My 'damaged' left eye has healed and completely returned to normal, something the doctor said was impossible. I have lost 60 pounds and seven pants sizes so far—I don't remember the last time my pant size was in the single digits! I am enjoying more energy and vitality than ever.

"The hardest part of the shift to plant-based was preparing food ahead and having the means to take it with me for meals on the go. What works for me is always being prepared with healthy meals made ahead and individually packaged in both the refrigerator and the freezer. With my crazy schedule I would never survive if I had to come home every night and figure out what to cook. I have purchased several containers that can go from freezer to microwave. I mainly cook on the weekends, and then have meals to take to work—stored in my great soup-size Thermos container—and ready to heat up for dinner when I get home. Another great thing is that since my husband is not a plant-based eater, many of my meals can be served to him with the addition of some grilled chicken, although as time goes by he is starting to eat a lot of my plant-based meals!

"My health crisis as well as my 'all-or-nothing personality' supported an overnight change to whole food, plant-based eating. After regaining my health and vitality I have started my own business sharing with others the wonderful benefits of a plant-based lifestyle. Thinking back to last year at this same time when my weight had spiraled out of control, my blood pressure was skyrocketing, and I suffered the retinal artery hemorrhage . . . I am an entirely new woman."

CHAPTER 13
Mastering Strength of Mind

What's the secret to mobilizing your mind for lifestyle change? What galvanizes the spark for transformation to become reality? Just as there are systems for food preparation, workplace readiness, and moving more, there are systems and strategies for the *inner* workings of lifestyle change. Dismantling old behaviors incompatible with the lifestyle changes you want—and building new ones that *are* compatible—can also be achieved with a step-by-step approach, unearthing you from old mental ruts and getting you into a new groove with your plant-based plan.

In this chapter, we'll examine the challenges of change. We'll take a closer look at the practical steps to transformation that you have been leveraging throughout this book—*become aware, set your intention, identify,* and *practice*—for they are the same tools you will implement for inner change. The conscious competence-learning model follows, explaining how the learning curve to a new lifestyle can play itself out and delivering reassurance for the sometimes rocky road of transition.

WHAT YOU EAT AFFECTS HOW YOU THINK

Research tells us that eating more fruits and vegetables improves mood, increasing your sense of optimism. Diets high in saturated fats and refined

---

sugars and low in fruits and vegetables have been found to reduce BDNF, the protein in the brain that we met in chapter 12, also believed to play a central role in mood states and depression.[1]

A daily intake of at least seven fruits or vegetables is associated with a meaningful increase in happiness and energy.[2] Those who eat more servings score themselves as significantly more optimistic and energetic than those who eat fewer.[3] You literally build a better outlook for change by what you eat.

CHANGE CHALLENGED?

A positive attitude can only get you so far—and motivation can be fickle. It is extremely helpful to understand what compels us to do what we do, why it can be hard to change, and why the process is so uneven. And why that's okay and how to deal with it. This calls for examining the underlying obstacles to change, implementing a system for revision, and respecting the process of transformation.

Habits vs. Practices

Habits can be a force for good or hold us back. A habit is something you do practically—or completely—without conscious thought. Actually, it's a good thing we have them. Can you imagine if every time you brushed your teeth or backed the car out of the garage you had to think through every step? Habits make life easier—unless they are bad habits, like grabbing junk food when we're stressed. Yet habits can be systematically dismantled and reconstructed to support you in creating healthy change.

When it comes to behavior change, I prefer the term *practices* to *habits*. It invites successful intervention and reminds us that habits are, after all, just things that we are used to doing—practicing—over and over again. Our affinity for routine compels us to repeat behaviors. Yet simply desiring different outcomes is not enough. Successful change requires examining the practices you already have in place, replacing them with new ones, and practicing *them* instead.

This extends to thinking practices, too. When entangled in my own personal struggle with weight, I discovered I not only had to address *what* I was eating, but I also needed to examine the practices of thinking that kept me caught in a loop of weight loss that was repeatedly followed by disheartening gain. Without addressing this internal element, I would not enjoy the success I relish today. If you have ever been frustrated in your attempts to make healthy change—thinking that you just don't have what it takes to mentally make the switch—I'm here to tell you that you do. All it takes is some innovation to reveal your secret inner strength.

When our best-laid healthy plans fall apart, we think we are weak-willed. Actually, this isn't true. Think about any endeavor that you have successfully achieved—securing a job, getting a degree, growing a garden, learning to drive, or running a 5K. These all take focus and strength of mind. If you have ever been able to drum up the discipline to do any such projects, you have what it takes. Your mind has tremendous strength and simply persists in what it knows best—your past practices. This is precisely your entry point for change: practicing new behaviors that are consistent with your new intentions.

Why Resolutions Fall Apart—and What to Do about It

We understand the problem, we discover the solution, and somehow the switch never proceeds quite as smoothly as we thought. Lapses happen—for all of us. Rather than letting it be your undoing, derailing you from the journey, simply understanding what's happening when you miss the mark changes the game for the better. Instead of abandoning your mission, you can turn backsliding around by making it your friend, implementing it as a tool to move you forward.

Realize that even the most welcome change is going to be met with some internal resistance. When you know, going in, that change—even for the better—is going to generate some discomfort, you put yourself at an advantage. The secret is learning to be present with this discomfort. Instead of it being your undoing, you leverage it as a springboard for your success. The uneasiness you experience when you deviate from your norm—your established practices—is completely normal. Our behaviors, right along with our bodies and brains, have a tendency to gravitate toward the status quo, kind of like the cruise control on your car, or your house thermostat. Maintaining internal stability—physiological homeostasis—also plays itself out in our unconscious attempt to maintain psychological equilibrium. Our innate resistance to change, even for the better, is a universal experience—the "inevitable escort of transformation."[4] Learning how to navigate this resistance will revolutionize your success.

Expecting backlash from within equips you in advance. Internal resistance is simply the red flag of change—the very change you seek. Be willing to negotiate with it. Start by becoming aware of how homeostasis shows up. It can appear in a variety of ways: as anxiety, even bickering with family or friends. It can manifest as negative self-talk and self-sabotage. You may find yourself thinking, "What's the point?" or feel stuck or bored, and need to feel safe by resurrecting old bad habits. As painful as they may be, they are familiar.

Rather than giving up or attempting to muscle your way through with willpower, there is another way. Keep pulling for change, but not without awareness and respect for the human predicament: that change is an uneven process. Be willing to take one step backward for every two forward, and vice versa. *Fighting* resistance always arms a war, even the one you may feel you are having with yourself. Compassion and understanding disarm it. It's just like an argument you might have with a friend. If you respond to a disagreement from a polarized, cemented position, pointing an accusing finger, it only leads to fiercer combat. If, on the other hand, you acknowledge the position of your opponent—for want of a better term—you calm the waters and create an entry point for resolution. You can start by telling your mind, "It's okay—I understand why you're unsettled!" Think of it as resistance training for your mind as you build more mental muscle.

You will also most likely encounter resistance from family or friends along the way. This may show up in overt or covert attempts to undermine your self-improvement. Recognize that this may simply be social homeostasis at work. When any part of the system changes, including social systems, everything else is going to be affected. Keeping this in mind—and realizing that these people probably aren't consciously wishing you harm—can make all the difference.

Some resistance challenges can lie deeper under the surface. Those self-generated can be particularly challenging to uncover, making them even more insidious. These, too, can be changed via the four steps we have been implementing throughout. Let's take a closer look at them.

FOUR STEPS TO TRANSFORMATION

Outfitted with an understanding of the reasons for resistance, let's take another look at the now familiar practical steps to change—*become aware, set your intention, identify,* and *practice*—as modeled with Susan, J.C., Nichole, Janice, and every successful story of transition throughout this book. These same steps give you a system for transforming underlying obstacles as well.

Then, I'll share with you some excellent examples from my clients of applying these steps.

Become Aware

The most basic of all beginnings is awareness of how your behaviors are getting you where you currently are. When you become aware of your repeated, habituated behaviors—and that includes practices of thinking—only then can you gain insight into how they may be holding you back and give you some choice about how to change them.

Clarify Your Intention

The next action is to set an intention. The word *intention* is somehow less intimidating than the word *goal*. It's positive and energetic. On the plant-based journey, your intention, the big picture, is to take your plate from plant-deficient to plant-predominant so that you can achieve your desired outcomes. From this broad view, become more specific about what you are going after. Your intention must be clear. Saying you want to be "perfectly healthy forever" is too vague. In contrast, "eating 90 percent whole food, plant-based" is specific. Clarity makes you more mentally poised for success by putting you in better inner alignment.

Identify Micro Changes

Identify the *micro changes* you need to make in order to fulfill your intention. These are the specific actions you need to take to get you from where you are to where you want to go. Specific actions—micro behaviors—taken one after another decide your health and dietary destiny. Mentally, establishing micro changes shifts what might seem overwhelming into smaller, doable tasks. These are always items that can be checked off a list. The goal of eating seven or more servings of vegetables and whole grains or starchy vegetables a day—as you saw in chapter 7—is a perfect example. Walking for forty-five minutes five times this week is another. Create simple charts for these specific behaviors and check them off every time you achieve them. This builds mental and emotional self-efficacy, confidence, and momentum.

No objective is too small. For example, let's say you establish the intention of walking every day. If you are currently engaged in no exercise other than jumping in and out of your car, and are struggling to connect your current state of fitness to any semblance of an exercise program, then going from zero to forty-five minutes a day is quite likely setting the bar too high. Start by committing to setting out your walking clothes every day for the next five days. When you've checked that micro change off your chart, the next week you can commit to putting on your walking clothes before or after work every day. Because these are all critical steps to actually completing a walk, they are positive behaviors—micro changes—worthy of recognition. They also increase the likelihood that you'll get out and take a walk. The next week, you only have one new micro change to make—actually going on a walk. For some this progression will be speedier. Find your own transition timeline. You want your actions to be compatible with your intention, and making doable micro changes is the easiest way to get there. They are your precise entry points for change.

Identifying specific dates to follow through on the micro changes provides a feedback loop by which you can measure your progress. Remember, behaviors change before they show up as results in improved health and weight loss. While staying mindful of your big picture boosts your journey, it is the specific behavior changes you make on a daily basis that carry you forward.

Practice!

Repeated practice forms new behavior patterns. Your choices become your habits, which in turn become your lifestyle. The same four steps apply to patterns of thinking and overcoming underlying obstacles, demonstrated beautifully by my clients Katherine and Dianna.

Case Study: Katherine

Frustrated in her attempts to follow through on her new healthy eating plan, Katherine came to me for help. She would go along just fine for a couple of weeks, enjoying her eating and workouts, and then for some inexplicable reason the food would fall apart. She'd find herself seriously sabotaging her best efforts, in her mind effectively obliterating all of the good practices she'd put in place. She was prepared with all the right foods—hunger wasn't the problem. But something kept aborting her healthy mission. To progress, she would need to uncover the hidden obstacle so she could address it with the four steps and break through the barrier to change.

I walked Katherine through a strategy that invited her to get under the surface of hidden resistance, thus delivering insights about behaviors. Several minutes into the process, I heard an audible gasp over the phone. I knew

Katherine had just experienced a moment of realization—*awareness*—of her hidden obstacle. Katherine's problem wasn't with her eating plan, exercise plan, or even her motivation. In a flash she realized that her new healthy lifestyle quite likely posed a threat—whether real or imagined—to her relationship with a very dear friend. A friend with whom she shared a history of weight struggles. They were also eating buddies. In that moment, she realized that unilaterally making the changes for healthy eating was upsetting the homeostasis of the friendship. Without illuminating this deep-seated yet overpowering conflict, Katherine would have been doomed to play out its repercussions over and over again, sabotaging her efforts at realizing her lifestyle dream.

With all the cards now on the table, she could effectively make some decisions over what to do about it. It would be necessary to negotiate her resistance to this problem, and we discussed her options about how to do just that. Her *intention* was to enjoy her workouts and food plan, while at the same time keep her friendship intact. It was clear to Katherine that she needed to *identify* a choice here—either support herself in healthy change, or back off so as not to rock the friendship boat. Or she could have an honest conversation with her friend about the problem, thus establishing a new *practice* of honesty in her friendship. Making this choice was essential for Katherine to move forward. Now, she could take effective action and stop getting in her own way. Without getting to the bottom of this underlying problem, she would have been destined to repeat the practice of self-sabotage.

In Katherine's situation, *awareness* of the pattern of repeated self-sabotage was essential before she could do anything about it. Clarifying her *intention*—to continue her healthy eating plan while keeping her friendship intact—allowed her to define her options. From there, *identifying* specific action and a date to follow through created a new behavioral *practice.*

READER TIP: MINDFUL AWARENESS GETS EASIER

"Your approach to living a healthy lifestyle involves not only food and exercise, but also a mindful awareness of choices and actions. It's easy to dismiss this component because most of us are focused on quick weight loss results, but those who do are missing out. Being mindful and aware of my choices and actions is exactly what I need when I go grocery shopping and feel tempted by candy bars at the checkout stand. It's exactly what I need when I think I'm too tired or too short on time to fix proper food. A quick rethink of the situation puts me right back on track—and it gets easier each time."

—Susan P.

Case Study: Dianna

Dianna, who came to me for help in losing weight, provides another example of how to work these four steps for successful outcomes.

Dianna told me that she had struggled for a long time with eating during the evening hours, even after a satisfying dinner. This was obviously getting in the way of her health and weight loss goals. First, we made certain that Dianna was eating enough throughout the day. This eliminated it as a driver of evening overeating. Soon we discovered that Dianna's after-dinner noshing had become a signal for her to transition to at-home activities. Quite quickly, it had become an established practice that had taken on a life of its own. What Dianna needed was something to mark the change from her busy day to evening activities that would replace her practice of eating more than she really wanted. To just try to halt the behavior—evening overeating—was not going to solve the problem. The practice of needing a transition activity was not the issue; the specific way she was meeting this need was.

Let's see how the steps play out in Dianna's story. Once Dianna became *aware* of and realized the real need—a transition activity—of the *intention* behind her after-dinner habit, the next steps were clear. We worked together to *identify* something else she could do to signal this evening shift. We found an exercise class that she had wanted to try, which she started attending two evenings out of the week right after dinner. On the other three days, her plan was to take a short walk immediately after dinner. Dianna made three important micro changes to the troublesome evening problem: 1) attend evening exercise class, 2) go on an evening walk, and 3) change her after-dinner environment. Removing herself from the environment that was reinforcing problematic practices helped Dianna obtain a new result.

Within two weeks of *practice*, these had become Dianna's new evening transition patterns, and she no longer struggled with the after-dinner problem as before. This is an example of how nonproductive practices can be dismantled and refurbished, via micro changes, with those compatible with your personal health goals. It may seem like an obvious solution. Yet without awareness of the true nature of her challenge, Dianna would have stayed locked in the behavior that was blocking her progress. Teasing apart the layers of current habits and replacing them with desired behaviors provides a system and a clear path to change.

INSIDE JOB

There's another factor that may be keeping you bound in a lesser life than the one you dream of—your thinking patterns.

Thoughts—Feelings—Actions—Results

Thinking patterns are the most insidious of all habituated practices, with their power to invisibly drive what we do. Understanding how to implement change at this level is arguably the single biggest thing that made success possible for me. The four steps can be applied here as well.

Mental mastery doesn't mean you're suddenly in control of your thoughts. Thoughts come unbidden, with a seeming life of their own, based on our experiences and a million connections made in our brain. They evoke feelings established during past experiences, initiating a set of ingrained patterns of behavior. And so, we keep getting the same results.

Autopilot can be a lifesaver. But when it hijacks your thoughts and pulls your behavior into a sinking spiral, there's definitely a downside. Thus, we need to interrupt the point between the emotional response and the ingrained behavior and replace it with *new* responses, giving you different results. You open the door to a whole new world of possibility when you start to see thoughts, impulses, and mood states as objects with changeable forms. It loosens their grip. This gives you a point of intervention for a different response than that to which you are habituated; it's an opportunity to take a fresh look at your experiences.

An example from my own struggles was the essential task of breaking out of cemented thought patterns about weight loss. With such a long history of failure when it came to weight management, I felt discouraged about once again embarking on the journey before I had even started. I brought a lot of baggage to the table in the form of negative associations, resulting in damaged self-efficacy, trepidation, and outright fear. What would be different this time? I knew to be successful in the way I really wanted I would have to navigate uncharted territory within. In practical terms, this is what I did to make the difference: I became willing to become *aware* of rising thoughts, the emotions that followed, and the response patterns that had become my practice. In the past, the negative thoughts and emotions about weight challenges had created a spiral of angst and fear that, hitched up with hunger and deprivation from dieting, drove eating behaviors that were in direct conflict with what I wanted. I made two new *intentions*. First, to start eating better. Second, to experience the discomfort of fear without following through on the urge to escape. I'd never thought of that before. Yet I found that the only way around the problem was to go right through the middle of it by practicing mindfulness meditation.

Mindfulness Meditation: Change Your Mind, Change Your Life

A mindfulness meditation practice—the intentional, accepting, and nonjudgmental awareness of the emotions, thoughts, and sensations occurring in the present moment[5]—created in me a new way to process them. This derailed the previous reaction patterns that kept me overweight. It delivered new results. It is reflected in the mindfulness exercise I implemented with Katherine for her breakthrough. And it can do the same for you.

Research underscoring the efficacy of mindfulness meditation to significantly augment the function of your prefrontal cortex—the command center of your brain—is rapidly on the rise.[6] This research shows mindfulness meditation can change regions in the brain involved in learning, memory, and emotion regulation,[7] and can reduce impulsivity.[8] Even brief periods of practice can be of benefit, serving as a quick and efficient strategy to counter depleted self-control during periods of low emotional resources and willpower reserves.[9] You will begin to see your attitudes more clearly, and come to identify which are helpful, which create difficulties, and what to do about them.

THE CONSCIOUS COMPETENCE LEARNING MODEL

Most of us experience an emotional learning curve when it comes to change. Realizing that this is a healthy and natural part of the process can be deeply comforting, and it enlightens and uplifts your journey. The Plant-Based Journey stages—Awakening through Champion—are reflected in what is known as the Conscious Competence Learning Model.[10,11] Enchantingly simple, this model describes a person's path from unawareness to mastery during the course of learning new skills, while acknowledging that there are emotional undercurrents to the process. Understanding the common emotions of each stage gives you the benefit of foresight.

We rarely have an appreciation for how much we will need to learn when undertaking something new. When we discover what we don't know about a subject, we can feel overwhelmed, become disheartened, and consider throwing in the towel. Acknowledging this helps you navigate some of the emotional ups and downs that can be part of the process. According to the Conscious Competence model, the levels we move through in the process of building competence in a new skill—such as the skills you are learning on the plant-based journey—are each accompanied by their own undercurrent of emotions.

Unconsciously Incompetent

Sometimes called blissful ignorance, this level means you are unaware that you lack a particular skill—or even that you need to learn it. Before contemplating the plant-based lifestyle, you may have been unaware of the problems posed by eating animal products and highly processed foods and that there is a different, health-building alternative. You may even have experienced denial about the usefulness of learning new skills for healthier meals. The Awakening process changed all that.

Consciously Incompetent

At this level, you become aware of the existence and relevance of a new skill, yet you can't do it very well. On the plant-based journey, this is represented by the Scout level, and it spills into your new skills practice as Rookie. You may occasionally feel disheartened by the effort it takes to plan and prepare. Yet you can reassure yourself that, while learning this skill might be difficult and frustrating right now, things will improve in the future. By making the commitment to learn and practice the new skill, you can move toward the "consciously competent" stage.

Consciously Competent

At this level you now know what to do, yet you still need to concentrate in order to perform. You've learned the basics—now it's practice, practice!—the single most effective way to move to the next stage. At this level, the model reminds you to value the skills that you've gained and appreciate that though the skills are not yet second nature or automatic—hallmarks of the Rookie—it's getting a lot easier. At this level, you know that you have acquired the skills and knowledge you need. You enjoy growing confidence.

Unconsciously Competent

The skill has become second nature. It seems so easy in contrast to where you started, and you might wonder what all the fuss was about early on. On the plant-based journey, this correlates to Rock Star and Champion. You are confident of success, without being compulsive about perfection. You understand that once you master one set of skills, it's important to learn more if you want to continue to advance your journey.

Bear in mind that you might feel uncomfortable during the consciously incompetent and consciously competent phases. But that's a good thing because it means you've moved out of your comfort zone—remember homeostasis and resistance—which is absolutely necessary on the journey to your desired lifestyle change. Being reminded of this helps. Look at it this way: If you are experiencing a little bit of discomfort, then you're probably doing something right. Unconscious competence can only be achieved through practice at the consciously competent stage. Rest assured that once you are at this ultimate desired destination, any feelings of discomfort simply fade away.

THE ROAD TO MASTERY

In making the leap from plant-based theory to plant-based living, one thing has proven successful over and over again, and you've met this idea before. Powered by the dual engines of keeping it simple and being prepared, *practice* is traction for the journey. Every eating event during the day—from a quick snack or a rushed lunch to commuter carry-on chow or a sit-down supper—is an opportunity to practice the plant-based lifestyle. That's all it is. A series of eating episodes that present you with another chance to make micro changes and exercise your skills. See it as practice rather than performance. Practice is how you get better at something. It's how you gain mastery, while taking the pressure of perfection off the table. When black belt masters go to the dojo, they say they are "going to practice." Even the baseball all-stars show up for batting practice. Practice is the raw material from which habits and success are built.

Given half a chance, your body's brilliant, inherent system of rejuvenation will restore you to radiant health. Implementing pragmatic steps for change, creating an environment of success via preparation, physical exercise, and flexing the muscles of mental mastery—along with a respect for the steps to conscious competence—equips you for success. Patience, understanding, and some compassion for yourself are the indispensable sojourners.

Along with the systems, stages, and steps for change, cultivate an adventurous energy around what you are doing. By all means, don't lose sight of the importance of enjoying what you eat. And never, ever lose your sense of humor. You may just become the healthiest, happiest person you know.

CHAPTER 14
Crowd-Pleasers and Can't Misses

Plant-based eating can often be *caught* even better than taught. Once family, friends, and the folks at the occasional potluck get a chance to try some delicious plant-based fare, you pique curiosity and win hearts. A focus on serving tasty fare will pay off in big dividends. These slightly fancier recipes are perfect for sharing at social events and potlucks, family gatherings, and special occasions—and for a grand slam at home, too.

QUICK RECIPES

If you're on the go and looking for quick recipes, keep an eye out for this symbol next to recipes! It only takes ten minutes to get these eats to your table or oven.

PREPARING PANS FOR BAKING

To bypass the use of oils to coat pans when baking, you have several options. Parchment paper—available at most supermarkets and reusable to an extent—can be used to line loaf pans and cover baking trays to create a nonstick surface. Silicone loaf pans, muffin trays, and mats placed atop baking sheets accomplish the same thing. Another technique that I've used quite a bit is to dip a finger in almond or sesame butter—it only takes a tiny amount—and spread a very thin film over the bottom of the pan. This works well in pie and bread pans.

BREAKFAST

PUMPKIN MUFFINS

This recipe is adapted from the Easy Pumpkin Muffins in The China Study Cookbook, *by LeAnne Campbell. Just like LeAnne, I use whole foods for sweetening when I can, and I decided to make this recipe using date cream—with excellent results. Sweet, moist, and delicious, these don't beg for even a hint of jam, though a dab of Sweet Bean Cream (page 203) is a perfect match—kind of like whipped cream on pumpkin pie.*

DATE CREAM
- 10 pitted Medjool dates (about 1 cup)
- ½ cup water

MUFFIN BASE
- 2 cups whole wheat pastry flour
- 1 teaspoon baking powder
- 1 teaspoon baking soda
- 1 teaspoon cinnamon
- 1 teaspoon allspice
- ½ teaspoon ginger
- ½ teaspoon nutmeg
- ½ teaspoon salt
- ½ (16-ounce) can pumpkin puree (about 1 cup)
- ¼ cup soured plant milk (see instructions on page 223)
- ⅓ cup applesauce
- ½ cup raisins
- ½ cup chopped walnuts (optional)

For the date cream:

1. Cover the pitted dates generously with water and soak for a couple of hours or overnight. Drain, saving the water to use as part or all of the ½ cup of water in the recipe. Add the soaked dates and the water to a food processor or blender. Blend to a rich paste.

For the muffin base:

1. Preheat the oven to 350 degrees.

2. Line a 12-cup muffin pan with paper liners (or use a silicone pan).

3. Mix together the dry ingredients in a large bowl.

4. In a separate bowl, combine the wet ingredients, including the date cream. Add to the dry ingredients until just mixed.

5. Fill the prepared muffin cups to the top and bake for 40–45 minutes, until the tops bounce back when lightly pressed. Muffins will be moist and flavorful.

6. Remove from the oven and let stand for 1–2 minutes, then remove the muffins from the pan and serve as is, with Sweet Bean Cream (page 203), or with your favorite jam. Store in an airtight container.

YIELD: About 10 muffins

CRISPY COCONUT WAFFLES ⊙

The slight bit of coconut flour in these waffles gives them a cake-like crumble; the brown rice flour adds incomparable crunch. No need for added sweetener in the batter—the natural sweetness of the coconut takes care of that. If waffles aren't your thing, the batter also makes wonderful pancakes.

  1 cup whole wheat pastry flour
  ⅓ cup coconut flour
  ⅓ cup brown rice flour
  ⅓ cup garbanzo flour
  ½ teaspoon salt
  1 tablespoon baking powder
  1 flax egg (see instructions on page 224)
  1 cup plant milk
½–⅔ cup water

1. Mix the dry ingredients in a large bowl.

2. Add the wet ingredients to the dry, including the flaxseed egg. Stir just until moistened.

3. Bake in a hot waffle iron, according to your model's instructions.

4. Serve topped with fresh fruit and maple syrup, or a spoonful of nondairy yogurt.

YIELD: 3 waffles, or about 12 pancakes

PANCAKES PRONTO ⓒ

This answers the question, "How do you make pancakes without milk or eggs?" These hotcakes are as fluffy as summer days are long. The secret is in the soured nondairy milk and mixing with a light hand, just enough to get the big lumps out and everything moist. In other words, stir as little as possible!

> 2 **cups whole wheat flour**
> 1 **tablespoon baking powder**
> ½ **teaspoon salt**
> 1½ **cups soured plant milk (see instructions on page 223)**
> ½ **cup applesauce or water**
> 1 **flax egg (see instructions on page 224)**

1. Mix the dry ingredients together in a large bowl.

2. Mix the wet ingredients in a medium bowl. Add to the dry mixture, folding the wet mixture in without overstirring—it should be a bit lumpy.

3. Heat a large griddle or nonstick pan over medium heat. Pour roughly ⅓ cupfuls of batter onto the griddle, and cook until the edges are slightly dried and bubbles forming on the top of the cakes start to pop. Flip with a spatula, and cook another minute or so until done.

4. Serve topped with fresh fruit and maple syrup. This also makes excellent waffles.

YIELD: About one dozen 4-inch pancakes or 3–4 waffles

NOTE

Often I'll switch out ¼ cup of the flour for brown rice flour, which adds an extra crunch.

BLACK BEAN POLENTA PIE

Ever since my first trip to Switzerland, I've been hooked on polenta. When hiking on a high alpine trail one day, my husband, Greg, and I turned a corner and happened upon a stone hut where a big, glorious golden vat of polenta was being stirred over an open fire. With my undying love for the combination of black beans and corn, this dish was an inevitable innovation. Though it has changed over the years, here is my most recent incarnation of this house favorite. With its three colorful layers—a golden polenta base, the black bean/bulgur layer in the middle, and the bright red salsa on top, along with the option of green guacamole for a fourth layer—this dish makes a beautiful presentation and has won the heart of many an omnivore dinner guest.

½   cup bulgur
1   cup vegetable broth
1   cup dry polenta
1   teaspoon cumin
½   teaspoon salt
3   cups water
2   cups frozen corn
1   medium sweet onion
2   teaspoons garlic powder
¼   cup plant milk
1   (14.5-ounce) can diced tomatoes (about 2 cups)
1   (15-ounce) can black beans (about 2 cups), rinsed and drained
2   teaspoons chili powder
2   teaspoons cocoa powder
1   teaspoon chipotle powder
1   cup salsa (mild or spicy, your choice)

1. Prepare a 9 x 13-inch baking dish.

2. Put the bulgur and vegetable broth in a medium bowl, stir, cover, and let sit for 3–4 hours, until the broth is absorbed into the bulgur. If you are in a hurry, you can cook the mixture in a rice cooker or on the stove instead. Set aside.

3. Preheat the oven to 350 degrees.

4. Place the polenta, cumin, salt, and water in a large saucepan and cook over medium heat, stirring or whisking every couple of minutes to prevent the mixture from getting lumpy or sticking to the bottom. Stir until the polenta has thickened enough that it doesn't settle back on the bottom of the pan when you stop stirring, about 10 minutes.

5. Stir the frozen corn (no need to thaw first) into the polenta and put a lid on the pot to heat the corn through (about 15 minutes). Turn off the burner and set aside.

6. While the corn is heating up in the hot polenta, dice the onion and place in a medium saucepan with the garlic powder and plant milk. Cook over medium heat, stirring, until the onion softens. Add the tomatoes, black beans, chili powder, cocoa powder, and chipotle powder to the onion mixture, then stir in the cooked bulgur.

7. Spread the polenta/corn mixture into the prepared pan, and smooth evenly with a spatula, pressing gently into the bottom of the pan.

8. Pour the black bean, bulgur, and tomato mixture on top of the polenta/corn and smooth. Pour the salsa over the black bean, bulgur, and tomato layer and distribute evenly.

9. Bake for 30 minutes. Cut into slices and serve, storing any leftovers in an airtight container in the refrigerator.

YIELD: 6-8 servings

NOTE

Serving Options: Serve with a bowl of fresh guacamole or dollop a spoonful on the top of each piece. Top with a sprinkling of chopped fresh cilantro. Alternatively, top with a dab of Cashew Cream (see note on page 196).

GAME-CHANGER CHILI

Just as in the Black Bean Polenta Pie (page 192), the bulgur here creates a meaty texture that pleases everyone from plantophiles to sworn omnivores. I like to serve Game-Changer Chili in large, wide bowls with golden chunks of Country Comfort Corn Bread (page 194) perched on top. Be prepared for everyone to ask for seconds.

   2 sweet onions
   1 red or yellow bell pepper

1½ cups bulgur

1 (14.5-ounce) can diced tomatoes (about 2 cups)

3 dates, soaked overnight and mashed into a paste

1 tablespoon chili powder

1 tablespoon smoked or regular paprika

1 tablespoon oregano

4 cloves garlic, pressed or chopped, or 2 teaspoons garlic powder

1 teaspoon chipotle powder

1 teaspoon adobo seasoning

Pinch of red pepper flakes (optional)

6 cups water

2 (14.5-ounce) cans kidney or red beans (about 4 cups), rinsed and drained

2–3 cups raw spinach, torn

1 cup cooked corn (optional)

Salt to taste

1. Chop the onions and bell pepper in a food processor, or dice with a knife.

2. Place the chopped onions and bell pepper, bulgur, tomatoes, dates, chili powder, paprika, oregano, garlic, chipotle powder, adobo seasoning, red pepper flakes, and water in a pressure cooker and cook under pressure for 7 minutes. Alternatively, you can also cook on the stove top for about 30 minutes, or until the bulgur is cooked through.

3. Stir in the beans, spinach, and corn, and let sit for about 5 minutes. Salt to taste. Serve in bowls.

YIELD: 4–6 servings

NOTE

If you don't have all of the seasonings, such as the chipotle and adobo, you can simply add more chili powder to taste. You can add them next time!

COUNTRY COMFORT CORN BREAD ⓖ

I recently made some changes to this favorite recipe that takes the delicious factor up a notch. Evidently, the tweaks took, because even though the recipe serves up nine average-size pieces of corn bread, my husband, Greg, and I nearly polished off the entire first batch between the two of us in one sitting. I served it atop big bowls of

Game-Changer Chili (page 193), a perfect companion. Take note—and make enough accordingly.

  1 cup whole wheat pastry flour
  1 cup yellow cornmeal
  2 teaspoons baking powder
  1 teaspoon baking soda
  ½ teaspoon salt
  1 cup soured plant milk, plus 2–3 tablespoons (see instructions on page 223)
  1 chia seed egg (see instructions on page 224)
  ½ cup unsweetened applesauce
  1 cup cooked corn

1. Preheat the oven to 400 degrees. Prepare an 8- or 9-inch square baking pan.

2. In a large bowl, combine the dry ingredients.

3. In a small bowl, combine the wet ingredients, then slowly add to the dry mixture, stirring just enough to mix. If it appears too dry and the flour isn't completely moistened, add more plant milk 1 tablespoon at a time accordingly.

4. Fold the corn into the batter, and pour the mixture into the prepared pan.

5. Bake for 25–30 minutes, until the surface is slightly browned and bounces back when you press it with your fingertips.

6. Let cool for a few minutes before serving.

YIELD: About 9 pieces

GOLDEN TURMERIC RICE Ⓖ

I've always considered raisins and rice to be perfect taste companions. This simple recipe brings the combination to dinner, spicing it up with nutritious turmeric powder. The addition of chickpeas creates a robust presentation, a filling main dish.

  2 cups short-grain brown rice
  1 (15-ounce) can chickpeas (about 2 cups), rinsed and drained
  2 teaspoons turmeric
  ⅓ cup raisins
  ½ teaspoon salt
  4 cups water

1. Place all the ingredients in a 1½-quart or larger rice cooker, stir, place the lid on the cooker, and cook according to your model's instructions.

2. Serve.

YIELD: 6–8 generous servings

NOTE

Add a side of salad and dinner is served!

MIYOKO'S SUN-DRIED TOMATO PESTO

Miyoko must be Japanese for "magic," for that's what my friend and plant-based chef Miyoko Schinner works in the kitchen. I asked Miyoko, a cookbook author many times over, if she would contribute a recipe or two to this section, and she delivered.

This is a very rich sauce due to the high fat content of the nuts—it's for special occasions!

- 1½ cups sun-dried tomatoes, dry (not oil-packed)
- 1   cup cashew cream (see note)
- 1½ packed cups basil leaves
- ½   cup pine nuts
- 6–10 cloves garlic
- 2–3 tablespoons white miso paste

1. Cover the sun-dried tomatoes with boiling water and let them soften for about 30 minutes while preparing the cashew cream.

2. When the tomatoes are soft, drain them well.

3. Combine all the ingredients in a food processor. Process until the desired texture is achieved, either completely smooth or a little chunky.

4. Serve tossed over pasta, whole grains, or vegetables.

YIELD: 2 generous cups

NOTE

To make cashew cream, use a blender to puree 1 cup of raw cashews with 3 cups of water until smooth.

||||||||||||||||||||||||||||||||||||||||||||||||||||||||||||||||||||||||||||||||||||||||||||||||||||||||||||||||||||||||||||||||||||||||||||||||||||||

LICKETY-SPLIT LASAGNA ©

||||||||||||||||||||||||||||||||||||||||||||||||||||||||||||||||||||||||||||||||||||||||||||||||||||||||||||||||||||||||||||||||||||||||||||||||||||||

Aka lazy cook's lasagna, this recipe shifts the paradigm on how long it takes to make what is traditionally a complex dish. The secret to speed is skipping the step of precooking the pasta. The only caveat is to make sure you don't skimp on the sauce, because the sauce provides the moisture that cooks into the pasta.

Don't let this lengthy-looking list of instructions fool you. It's simply breaking down the layers for ease of building your lasagna. I like to assemble this the day before I'll be serving it. It gets the flavors synergizing and the noodles get a head start on soaking up the moisture in the sauce for cooking.

  2 (7-ounce) packages seasoned baked tofu, thawed and squeezed to drain excess moisture

  2 (25-ounce) jars marinara or pasta sauce

 12 whole grain lasagna noodles (about one 12-ounce package)

  2 (10-ounce) bags frozen spinach, cooked and drained

  2 (4-ounce) cans sliced mushrooms, drained

1. Preheat the oven to 350 degrees.

2. Shred the tofu into bite-size pieces, either by hand or by pulsing in a food processor with the "S" blade.

3. Spread about 1½ cups of the sauce over the bottom of a 9 x 13-inch lasagna or casserole dish. Press 4 pieces of the dry pasta side by side into the sauce, and cover with another ½ cup of the sauce to create a thin layer on top of the noodles.

4. Scatter 1 cup of the crumbled tofu over the top of the sauce, then spread 1 cup of the spinach in a layer, then 1 cup of the sliced mushrooms.

5. Add 1 cup of the sauce on top, then press another 4 pieces of the dry pasta side by side, and cover with another ½ cup of the sauce.

6. Scatter the remaining crumbled tofu over the top, cover with the rest of the spinach, then cover with the remaining mushrooms. Spread another cup of the sauce over everything, press another 4 pieces of the dry pasta side by side, and cover with another ½ cup or more of the sauce, so all is covered.

7. Cover with parchment paper and seal the pan with aluminum foil. Bake for about 50 minutes, until cooked through and bubbling.

YIELD: 8 servings

NOTE

For a cheesier tasting lasagna, you can layer in ¼ cup of Nutty Plant Parmesan (page 206) after each layer of mushrooms, finishing with another ¼ cup on top. Olives also make a great addition.

PORTOBELLO POT ROAST

This recipe came to me as a happy surprise from my friend Jim Presentati. I first met Jim on our favorite mountain biking trail. Soon after he told me his phenomenal plant-based success story (see page 70). Jim raved about the "absolutely delicious portobello mushroom pot roast" that his wife, Kathy, makes. The next time I saw him, he mentioned it again. Time to investigate! When Kathy graciously sent me her recipe, I couldn't help but think it was a perfect match for this section of the book. Who doesn't know and love pot roast? The portobellos make the perfect savory swap-out and create a whole new gustatory experience. Here is my version, adapted from Kathy's recipe, with just a tweak or two.

- ½ cup white wine (you can also try red—I've even made this with sake), divided
- 4 large portobello mushrooms, sliced into ¾-inch pieces
- 1 large onion, sliced
- 2 cloves garlic, pressed
- 3 tablespoons flour
- 1 teaspoon rubbed sage
- 1 teaspoon dried basil
- 2–3 cups vegetable broth, divided
- 4 potatoes, quartered
- 4 carrots, cut into 3-inch pieces
   Salt and freshly ground black pepper or lemon pepper, to taste
- 2 teaspoons vegetarian Worcestershire sauce
- 1 sprig fresh rosemary
- 3–4 sprigs fresh thyme

1. Preheat the oven to 350 degrees.

2. In a large saucepan, heat ¼ cup of the wine and add the portobello mushroom slices. Allow them to cook through and brown a bit—you'll need to keep moving them around and turning them—and then remove from the pan and set aside.

3. Add the remaining ¼ cup wine to the pan and add the onion and garlic. Caramelize the onions by stirring them until they wilt and begin to brown. Remove the onions from the pan and set aside.

4. Mix the flour, sage, and basil together in a small bowl. Stir in ¼ cup of the broth to create a paste, and pour the mixture into the same pan you used for the mushrooms and onions. While stirring constantly over medium heat, very slowly add the rest of the broth so that you create a gravy or sauce.

5. When the mixture just starts to boil, turn the heat off and add any additional seasonings you prefer. (Kathy suggests parsley and pepper.)

6. Add the potatoes, carrots, salt and pepper, and Worcestershire sauce to the gravy mixture. If more liquid is needed to keep the vegetables from drying out, add more broth.

7. Add the mushrooms and onions to the mixture and ladle into a large ceramic or glass pot or casserole dish with a lid, layering in the sprigs of rosemary and thyme. Place the lid on and put into the oven and bake for 1 hour. Remove from the oven and serve hot.

YIELD: 4 servings

NOTE

ALTERNATE COOKING OPTIONS:
- If you have a large, heavy pot such as a Dutch oven that can go from cooktop to oven, you can prepare the entire dish in that fashion, as Kathy does.
- Assemble everything in a big pot on the stove or pressure cooker and cook until the vegetables are done. The flavor pizzazz provided by searing the mushrooms, onions, garlic, and gravy is compromised somewhat. Yet if you're pressed for time, each variation is delicious.

TACOS IN NO TIME ©

These make a filling, anytime meal. I've included directions here for making a single serving, as they make a great quick lunch. You can also serve two or three per person with a side salad and you're all set for dinner!

One 5½-inch corn tortilla
¼   cup fat-free refried beans

¼ **cup cooked brown rice or corn**
1 **tablespoon finely chopped sweet onion**
1 **tablespoon salsa**

1. Warm the tortilla briefly in a pan on the stove, or in the microwave.

2. Warm the beans and rice or corn in a pan on the stove or in a bowl in the microwave.

3. Spread the beans over the tortilla, then spread the rice or corn over the beans. Top with the onion and salsa.

4. Fold in half and serve.

YIELD: 1 taco

NOTE

You can also assemble everything cold and then pop the whole taco into the oven or microwave to quickly heat it. However, the corn tortillas tear easily if you try to fold them cold, so I like to warm them first.

SPEEDY BURRITOS ◉

A meal unto themselves, these burritos are delicious straight out of the oven, or wrap and store them in the fridge or freezer for on-the-go fare later. Food for Life makes a good sprouted grain burrito shell with no added fat.

⅓ **cup cooked short-grain brown rice**
    One 12-inch whole grain burrito shell
⅓ **cup black or pinto beans, rinsed and drained**
⅓ **cup cooked corn**
¼ **cup salsa**
2 **tablespoons finely chopped sweet onion**

1. Preheat the oven to 375 degrees.

2. Spread the rice on the shell, leaving about a ½-inch margin for rolling.

3. Spread the beans and corn over the rice, then layer the salsa over the beans.

4. Sprinkle the onion over the top. Gently press all the ingredients with a fork to compress slightly. This will help the burrito hold together when eating.

5. Pull one side of the shell over the ingredients to cover two-thirds of the wrap.

6. Fold the two ends of the burrito in by about one-third, creating an envelope.

7. Starting with the original folded edge, incorporating the enveloped ends, roll the burrito into a tube.

8. Wrap the burrito in a piece of parchment paper.

9. Place the paper-wrapped burrito on a baking sheet and bake for 10–15 minutes, depending on how warm your ingredients were to start with.

10. Serve topped with any of your favorites: diced avocado or guacamole, more salsa, or cashew cream.

YIELD: 1 burrito

NOTE

You can make these in large batches and place the paper-wrapped burritos in a plastic bag in the refrigerator or freezer. To warm up frozen burritos, simply increase the baking time until the burrito is warm. From the fridge, you might need to bake for 20 minutes; thawed from the freezer, about 30 minutes. You could also microwave these in about 2 minutes.

DRESSINGS, SAUCES, AND TOPPERS

‖‖‖
SWEET AND SOUR DRESSING ⓠ
‖‖‖

*This is my go-to low-fat dressing for salads, steamed vegetables, and
Buddha Bowls (page 112).*

- 6 tablespoons white balsamic vinegar
- 2 tablespoons wet mustard of choice
- 2 tablespoons maple syrup

1. Shake all the ingredients together in a jar. Taste, and adjust the amounts of
mustard or maple syrup as desired.

2. Store in the refrigerator.

YIELD: About ½ cup

‖‖‖
TAHINI-LEMON SAUCE ⓠ
‖‖‖

*If you've ever eaten Middle Eastern food, you'll recognize and love
these flavors.*

- ½–1 cup water
- ½ cup raw sesame tahini
- 1 clove garlic, crushed, or ½ teaspoon garlic powder
- ½ teaspoon salt or yellow miso
- 3 tablespoons lemon juice

1. Blend all the ingredients, starting with ½ cup of the water. Check the consistency,
and add more water, if desired, to thin.

2. Store in the refrigerator.

YIELD: 1¼–1½ cups

NOTE

To vary the flavor, add ¼ cup plain, unsweetened nondairy yogurt to the finished sauce.

MBEGU'S SPICY AFRICAN PEANUT SAUCE ⊙

Mbegu is Swahili for "seed." It is also the name of the first elephant Greg and I adopted in Kenya. I named this sauce, inspired by multiple delicious meals we were served in Africa, after her. This is what makes the African Buddha Bowl (page 113) African!

- 1 (14.5-ounce) can diced tomatoes
- ½ cup finely chopped onion
- 2 cloves garlic, crushed, or 1 teaspoon garlic powder
- ¾ cup liquid from drained tomatoes and/or vegetable broth, divided
- ½ teaspoon cumin
- ½ teaspoon cilantro
- ½ teaspoon salt
- 3 tablespoons peanut butter

1. Drain and finely chop the tomatoes, setting the liquid aside. Put the onion, garlic, and ¼ cup of the vegetable broth and/or liquid from the tomatoes in a medium saucepan and cook over medium heat until the onions are translucent.

2. Add the seasonings and stir, continuing to cook. Add the tomatoes, peanut butter, and remaining ½ cup broth, and heat through. The sauce will be slightly chunky from the tomatoes, yet fluid enough to use as a sauce.

3. Serve immediately over grains or vegetables or store in the refrigerator.

YIELD: About 2 cups

SWEET BEAN CREAM ⊙

This adds sweetness and staying power to breakfast biscuits, steamy bowls of grains, pancakes, waffles, and muffins. Cannellini beans are so mild flavored that they are extremely versatile in cooking—and thanks to the aromatic addition of the orange, vanilla, and cardamom, I guarantee no one will suspect there are beans in this light, delicious treat.

- 6 large Medjool dates, pitted
- ¼ cup orange juice

¼ cup water

1 (15-ounce) can cooked cannellini beans, rinsed and drained (about
   2 cups)

1 tablespoon raw almond butter

1 tablespoon orange zest

1 teaspoon vanilla bean paste or vanilla extract

½ teaspoon cardamom powder

1. Soak the dates in the orange juice and water for a few hours or overnight.

2. Place the soaked dates, including the orange juice and water, and remaining ingredients in a food processor or blender. Process until you have a fluffy sweet consistency. Add more water if desired to thin.

3. Store covered in the refrigerator.

YIELD: About 2 cups

NOTE

Alter the sweetness by adjusting the amount of dates. To lessen richness, reduce the almond butter. If you're in a hurry, you can probably skip soaking the dates by cooking them with the orange juice and water in a pan on the stove for a few minutes to soften.

CRANBERRY SAUCE WITH DATES AND ORANGES ⓠ

This sugar-free version of a holiday favorite has been a hit 100 percent of the times that I've served it, and has been one of the most popular recipe downloads from my blog. Buy extra cranberries when they are in season and store them in the refrigerator so that you can make this all year long. It's great for topping oatmeal and pancakes, or spread in sandwiches.

8 Medjool dates, pitted
   Juice from 1 orange

¼ cup water

1 (12-ounce) bag fresh cranberries (about 2½ cups)

1 tablespoon orange zest

1. Soak the dates in the orange juice for a few hours or overnight.

2. In a high-powered blender or food processor, blend the dates with the juice and the water.

3. Put the date mixture in a large pot with the cranberries. Cook over high heat for 5 minutes, then reduce the heat to low and cook for about 15 minutes. Add more water as needed so the mixture stays liquid though dense, like thick, chunky applesauce. Remove from the heat.

4. Let cool and store in the refrigerator. Serve as you would any cranberry sauce: with holiday dinners, or on cooked whole grains, mashed potatoes, your morning oatmeal, or to perk up a sandwich.

YIELD: About 2 cups

NOTE

If you're in a hurry, you can probably skip soaking the dates. If you do, cook them for a few minutes longer to soften.

APPLE VINAIGRETTE ⓒ

This is a light, sweet dressing perfect for salads or steamed vegetables, created by my friend Miyoko Schinner. She says that any crisp, sharp apple works beautifully in this recipe.

1 Braeburn, Granny Smith, or other crisp apple, cut into small chunks
1 small onion or ¼ large onion
Juice of 3–4 lemons
2 tablespoons champagne vinegar
1 tablespoon maple syrup
1 tablespoon Dijon mustard
Salt and freshly ground black pepper, to taste

1. Puree all the ingredients in a blender until smooth. Add salt and pepper to taste.

2. Store in an airtight container in the refrigerator.

YIELD: About 1 cup

NUTTY PLANT PARMESAN ⓠ

There are many options for plant-based parmesan these days. Here's my spin! You can increase or decrease the proportion of nuts as desired.

- 1 cup nutritional yeast
- ¾ cup raw cashews, almonds, walnuts, or pine nuts
- ¼ teaspoon salt
- ¼ teaspoon garlic powder or smoked paprika (optional)

1. Grind all the ingredients together in a food processor or blender, being careful to just grind until crumbly. If you overblend, it will become nut butter!

2. Serve sprinkled on vegetables, grains, pasta with or without marinara, baked potatoes, salads, chili—you name it.

YIELD: About 1½ cups

LIME CHIPOTLE CHICKPEAS ⓠ

I'm a huge fan of the versatile chickpea, aka garbanzo bean. The beans soak in a simple marinade, adding wonderful flavor. They can either be kept in the fridge to scoop into salads or for a side dish, or roasted in the oven, where they dry so that you can pop them into a baggie for convenient travel. I always double this because they keep well—and go fast.

- 2 (15-ounce) cans chickpeas (about 4 cups)
- 2 teaspoons onion powder
- 1 teaspoon oregano
- 1 teaspoon chipotle powder
- ½ teaspoon garlic powder
- 2 tablespoons lime juice
- 2 tablespoons balsamic vinegar
- 2 tablespoons tamari
- 1 teaspoon maple syrup

1. Rinse and drain the beans, and set aside.

2. Mix all the other ingredients in a large bowl, creating a marinade. Add the chickpeas and stir to coat.

3. Chill for a couple of hours in the refrigerator, occasionally stirring to mix the marinade through.

YIELD: About 4 cups

NOTE

TO CREATE THE ROASTED VERSION:

1. Preheat the oven to 400 degrees and line a shallow baking pan with parchment paper.
2. After marinating the beans, strain out the marinade, and spread the beans in a single layer on the baking sheet.
3. Roast for about 30 minutes. Keep an eye on the beans so that they don't dry out or burn.

DESSERT

MANDARIN CHOCOLATE ICE CREAM

Reminiscent of a favorite childhood dessert, this recipe requires a food processor or high-powered blender to prepare. It's also the easiest dessert to make!

- 3 frozen ripe bananas, cut into 1-inch chunks
- 3 tablespoons cocoa powder
- ¾ cup plant milk (see note)
- ½–1 teaspoon of orange extract, to taste

1. Pulse all the ingredients in a food processor or high-powered blender, pressing the contents down or mixing in frozen banana chunks as needed.

2. Pour all ingredients into a shallow container with a lid (I use sandwich size) and store covered in the freezer until set, about 4 hours. Scoop and serve.

3. You can also serve immediately, without freezing, as a soft-serve ice cream.

YIELD: 3 servings

NOTE

MILK NOTE: You can add more or less milk depending on the consistency desired. This recipe is very forgiving.

RICE COOKER BAKED APPLES

This dessert came out of a hankering for baked apples and desire for convenience. I don't know where the vision came from, but this method makes creating soft, sweet baked apples as easy as it gets!

- 2–4 Granny Smith apples (depending on how many apples you can fit in your rice cooker)
- 2–3 tablespoons raisins
  Sprinkle of cinnamon

1. Core the apples and place in the rice cooker without stacking them on top of each other. Press the raisins and cinnamon into the cored center of the apples. Pour about ½ inch of water into the rice cooker, and cook according to your model's instructions.

2. Check about every 15 minutes so you don't overcook or burn the apples. If all of the water evaporates, add more.

3. Serve warm in bowls as is, or topped with Mandarin Chocolate Ice Cream (page 208). On occasion, I'll cook them in the morning to sit atop waffles.

YIELD: 2–4 baked apples

NO SUGAR, NO OIL PECAN APPLE CRISP

From Miyoko Schinner, this makes a scrumptious, easy, and healthy dessert to follow a Sunday supper.

  6 Medjool dates, pitted
  ¾ cup water
  4 large or 5 medium crisp apples (ex: Fuji, Gala, Pippin, Granny Smith)
1½ teaspoons cinnamon, divided
  ¼ teaspoon nutmeg
  1 teaspoon vanilla extract
  1 cup raw pecans
  ½ cup raisins

1. Preheat the oven to 375 degrees. Prepare a 6 x 9-inch baking dish.

2. Soak the dates in the water for an hour or more. Puree the dates and water in a blender until creamy.

3. Cut or dice the apples into ½-inch chunks.

4. In a medium saucepan, combine the apples, date puree, 1 teaspoon of the cinnamon, nutmeg, and vanilla extract. Cover and bring to a simmer. Turn down the heat and continue simmering, stirring frequently, until the apples are hot and enrobed in a sauce.

5. Transfer the apples to the prepared dish.

6. In a food processor, combine the pecans, raisins, and remaining ½ teaspoon cinnamon. Process until pulverized and the mixture is crumbly. There should not be distinct pieces of raisins or pecans, but an integrated, crumbly mixture. Sprinkle over the apples.

7. Bake for 30–40 minutes, until the topping is browned and the apples are tender. If desired, serve with some nondairy whipped topping or ice cream.

YIELD: 6 servings

COLLEEN HOLLAND'S DOUBLE CHOCOLATE CHERRY TRUFFLES

My dear friend Colleen Holland, cofounder of VegNews *magazine, created these truffles for a mutual friend's birthday—and I've been a fan ever since. They taste like a walnut-fudge brownie, with hints of cherry and vanilla. I hope Colleen makes them for my next birthday . . . hey, a girl can dream!*

> 3 cups walnuts
> ½ cup cacao powder
> 1 teaspoon vanilla bean powder
> ½ teaspoon cinnamon
> ¼ teaspoon salt
> 15 soft Medjool dates, pitted (about 1½ cups)
> ½ cup dried cherries
> ¼ cup cacao nibs
> **Chopped walnuts, shredded coconut, or crushed cacao nibs, for dusting**

1. Place the walnuts, cacao powder, vanilla powder, cinnamon, and salt in a food processor. Process until the nuts are finely chopped but not powdered. While the food processor is running, slowly add the dates one at a time until well combined.

2. Lightly pulse the food processor while adding the cherries and cacao nibs. The cherries should remain in pieces.

3. Roll the dough into 1-inch truffles and roll in the chopped walnuts, shredded coconut, or crushed cacao nibs. Store in the refrigerator or gift to a special person in your life!

YIELD: 24 truffles

BERRYLICIOUS FRUIT TART

The first time I tasted these was at an Iron Chef *competition, where I had been asked to serve on the celebrity judge panel. Given an assortment of surprise ingredients and only twenty minutes to prepare, Chef AJ swept the desserts round with this entry—not surprising because for years Chef AJ was the executive pastry chef at Santé Restaurant in Los Angeles.*

CRUST

- 1 cup gluten-free oats
- 1 cup raw walnuts
- 1 cup unsweetened coconut
- 12 ounces pitted dates (about 1½ cups)
- 2 tablespoons lime juice plus zest of 2 limes

FILLING

- 8 ounces (about 2 cups) hulled strawberries
- 8 ounces (about 2 cups) Fuyu persimmons (see note)
- 4 tablespoons chia seeds
- 2 pounds (about 5 cups) fresh mixed berries (blackberries, blueberries, raspberries)

Shredded coconut, for garnish

For the crust:

1. In a food processor fitted with the "S" blade, process the oats, walnuts, and coconut into a flour. Add the dates and process until the mixture clumps and you can form a ball, adding more dates, if necessary. Then add the lime juice and zest. If the mixture becomes too wet, knead in more oats and coconut by hand.

2. Press the dough into a 10-inch fluted tart pan. Place in the freezer while preparing the filling.

For the filling:

1. In a blender, blend the strawberries and persimmons. Then add the chia seeds and blend again.

2. Add the mixed berries to a large bowl. Pour the strawberry/persimmon mixture over the mixed berries and stir gently.

To assemble:

1. Pour the filling into the crust in the tart pan.

2. Sprinkle with the shredded coconut and serve.

YIELD: 8–12 servings, depending on how you cut it!

NOTE

PERSIMMON NOTE: If persimmons are out of season, use 1 pound of strawberries. If they aren't sweet enough, add a few dates to sweeten.

ONWARD!

As a teacher, I find it hard to let go of my students at the end of the year. It is no different here, with you, in the final pages of this book. And just as with my students, I'm here to support you as you continue on your adventure, helping you build upon your progress, troubleshoot challenges, and celebrate your wins.

Becoming a plant-based eater is a journey—thus the title of this book. Changing your lifestyle may be difficult at times, but it can feel impossible if you hold yourself to a standard of perfection. Black-and-white thinking rarely moves you in the direction you want to go long term. Setbacks are bound to happen in the nonlinear reality of life.

Perfectionism should not be confused with striving for excellence. The latter positively energizes your reach for greater heights on the tree of doing your best; the former just keeps you in fear of falling off. Perfectionism comes with pain and shame as companions, which drive you to comfort coping rather than inspiring you to improve. In contrast, self-compassion and building on the positive do inspire you to improve. Real life calls for flexibility and "perfect enough." Avoid obsessing about food group balance, the size of your plate, the number of meals you eat, chewing each bite a certain number of times, or any other of a number of ways we can get distracted from the cause: eating more whole plant foods and less of everything else. Cultivate the attitude and mind-set of possibility, joyous anticipation, and opportunity. This will invite you to move forward with a spirit of adventure.

Take charge by being fully ready for whichever transition style works best for you. Just prepare, keep it simple, and go. Aim for more of the foods you envision on your ideal plate and less of the others. Pick your priority foods to pass on and up your plant content accordingly. To avoid getting lost in the gray area, be specific about incremental goals. Remember, simplicity rules, and sticking to a few favorite choices is all you need at the outset. Continue to grow the presence of whole plant foods on your plate so that everything else is side-dished, then crowded out. With intention and practice, soon you'll have so many go-tos and systems in place that the elimination rounds will be easy.

Make it a priority to find and make foods you like. The time investment to build your short list of front-runners will pay off big-time by keeping you well fed from day one as you expand your plant-based repertoire. While befriending your favorites, don't be shy about venturing into new taste territory. There will be a little trial and error and "fail yourself forward," as there is in any worthwhile venture.

Understand the value of staying connected to your "why," and the benefit of bonding with something bigger than yourself. While you are your own best support system, associate with others who are aspiring to the same ideal. Nourish the critical practices of physical activity and mental mastery that move your cart forward—juice for the journey. Avail yourself of the treasure of resources you'll find online at www.theplantbasedjourney.com, where you can also find a contact form to send me messages about your questions, concerns, and triumphs.

According to the research, there are distinct commonalities among individuals who achieve successful lifestyle change:[1]

- **Their personal reasons for changing—the "whys"—are clear.**
- **They acquire the skills necessary for change.**
- **They take ownership of the specific goals and methods they implement.**
- **They identify and address inner obstacles, the underlying barriers such as inner resistance and any self-efficacy mismatch.**
- **They engender support, accountability, and follow-through.**

If these look familiar, it is because these same salient points are reflected in the five stages of the plant-based journey, from Awakening through Champion. Once you set foot on the journey, and integrate these principles into your lifestyle, you'll enjoy an instant improvement, delivering to you extraordinary well-being and an unprecedented exuberance for living. Keep this book within reach as a resource for your adventure. Let it help you navigate change and give you direction, encouraging you as you discover your own personal pathway on the plant-based journey. *Avanti!*

APPENDICES

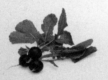

RESOURCES

For a rich reserve of lists and resources—everything from the scientific research to support systems, access to endless plant-centered recipes, food prep tips, and books that educate and inspire—go to www.theplantbasedjourney.com and navigate to Resources.

SHOPPING LIST

This shopping list, based on the contents of my own refrigerator and pantry, will get you started stocking your own plant-based kitchen. It is not necessary to rush out and procure everything on this list, by any means! Let your plant food arsenal grow right along with plantifying foods you are already familiar with and the templates and recipes you start to make. For a downloadable version, see Resources at www.theplantbasedjourney.com. There you will also find other helpful tutorials, including tips for cooking beans and grains.

The most economical way to procure beans, legumes, whole grains, dried fruits, nuts, and seeds is to buy in bulk, often available at natural foods stores. There is an extensive assortment of plant-based food items available online at specialty websites such as bulkfoods.com, vitacost.com, and amazon.com. To save on produce, shop the farmers' market, where you can often stock up for lower prices than the supermarket. In season, you can buy extra and freeze for later use.

VEGETABLES

acorn squash	celery	parsley
arugula	cilantro	portobello mushrooms
baby spinach	dried shiitake	red potatoes
bok choy	mushrooms	romaine lettuce
broccoli	garlic	sweet onions
Brussels sprouts	green beans	tomato salsa
butternut squash	green cabbage	yams
carrots	kale	Yukon gold potatoes

FRUIT

apples (fresh and dried)	bananas	oranges
apricots (fresh and dried)	Calimyrna figs	peaches
	cherries	plums
	Medjool dates	raisins

BULK DRIED FOODS

BEANS AND LEGUMES

black beans
chana dal
chickpeas
dried split pea flakes
French lentils
green split peas
kidney beans
orange lentils
pinto beans
red beans
red lentils
yellow split peas

GRAINS

Arrowhead Mills Organic Oat Bran Pancake and Waffle Mix

black rice
brown jasmine rice
brown rice cereal
bulgur
corn flour
cornmeal
old-fashioned rolled oats
pasta (whole grain, quinoa, etc.)
polenta
quick-cooking rolled oats
short-grain brown rice
shredded wheat cereal
whole oat groats
whole wheat pastry flour

BREAD

whole wheat bread
corn tortillas
sprouted cinnamon raisin bread
sprouted grain burrito wraps
sprouted grain sesame bread
whole grain tortillas
whole wheat lavash

FLOUR

brown rice flour
coconut flour
garbanzo flour
stone-ground whole wheat flour
whole corn flour
whole wheat pastry flour

FROZEN FOODS

bananas	kale	spinach
blueberries	mango	sprouted grain burrito wraps
cherries	mixed vegetables	veggie burgers
corn	peas	

CANNED/PACKAGED FOODS

black beans	garbanzo beans/ chickpeas	mushrooms
cannellini beans	kidney beans	olives
diced tomatoes	marinara sauce	soup cups
		tomato sauce

BAKING INGREDIENTS

applesauce
baking powder
baking soda
brown sugar

carob powder
cocoa powder
cornmeal
cornstarch

date sugar
En-R-G egg replacer
vanilla powder or
  extract

SEASONINGS AND CONDIMENTS

apple cider vinegar
brown rice vinegar
chipotle powder
cinnamon
cumin seeds and
  powder
curry vindaloo powder
dill

garlic powder
ketchup
mango chutney
nutritional yeast flakes
onion flakes
smoked paprika powder
sweet balsamic vinegar
sweet chili sauce

tamari
turmeric powder
vegetable broth
vegetarian seasoning
  (like Bill's Best
  Chik'nish Seasoning)
wet mustard
white balsamic vinegar

OTHER

cashews
chia seeds
flaxseeds
jam

maple syrup
oat milk
peanut butter
plain unsweetened
  soy milk

raw almond butter
raw tahini
sunflower seeds
walnuts

PLANT-BASED FAQS

Some regular questions emerge when it comes to transitioning to plant-based eating. It helps to have some responses prepared for the most common, so that you are better able to address the questions you may have, as well as those asked by others. Brief responses are usually best, followed by an offer to refer further reading should the questioner show interest. We'll briefly address a couple of the most common questions here. For deeper study on plant-based nutrition, see the Resources at www.theplantbasedjourney.com for a list of recommended books.

Q: Can you get all the protein you need from a 100 percent plant-based diet?

A: A varied, whole plant foods diet delivers nutrition perfectly suited to your needs—*inclusive* of protein. What we call "protein" is actually a functional assembly of the building blocks of protein, known as amino acids. *Amino acids are exactly the same wherever you find them*, whether they come from a beef steak or a beefsteak tomato. In whatever form you ingest protein, your body breaks it down into these original, individual building blocks—amino acids—and pools them to assemble as required. It maintains its own temporary storage of amino acids, working with those delivered by the different foods you eat throughout the day to produce just the right amounts and ratios that you need.

As far back as 1971 myths about amino acid shortages and food combining were put to rest by researchers in protein nutrition, stating that protein requirements can be easily met with a plant-based diet[1]—without the need to mix, match, or meticulously combine plants in some sort of science-project-style assembly for "complete" protein. Every plant that provides protein—which includes all vegetables, grains, legumes, nuts, and seeds—contains all of the essential amino acids that are needed by humans. Different plants may have higher percentages of some of the amino acids and lower percentages of others, but it doesn't matter for those who eat even the simplest variety of plant foods. Your body in its wisdom combines them for you. *The Journal of the American Dietetic Association*[2] emphatically states that a whole food, plant-based diet can meet all of our protein needs, and that eating a variety of plant foods throughout the day more than assures us of adequate protein intake. An exhaustive analysis of protein provided by plant foods in the *American Journal of Clinical Nutrition*[3] concludes, "Consumers do not need to be at all concerned about amino acid imbalances when the dietary amino acid supply is from the plant-food proteins that make up our usual diets. Mixtures of plant proteins can be fully adequate for meeting human requirements." As long as you are eating sufficient calories and are not eating a diet that is 100 percent fruit—or high in refined, processed foods—you are getting sufficient protein.

Back to the "where do you get your protein?" question. As an example, let me walk you through a protein analysis of some of the items you'd have found on my plate yesterday. Keeping the RDA for protein[4,5] in mind—0.36 grams per pound of body weight for men and women—my personal protein RDA comes out to about 49 grams. I easily obtain more than this by simply eating the following as I might on a typical day: 1½ cups of oatmeal (9 grams), 1 tablespoon flaxseed (1 gram), 1 cup black beans (15 grams), 2 cups raw spinach (1 gram), 1 cup brown rice (5 grams), 1 large stalk broccoli (7 grams), 1 medium potato (3 grams), 2 cups steamed kale (4 grams), and 1 cup lentil soup (10 grams).

I've even overshot my 49-gram protein RDA—and that doesn't include every incidental eaten throughout the day. Filling in the rest of the day's energy requirements with fruits, vegetables, possibly more starchy vegetables, and whole grains easily tips me into the balance of more than sufficient protein.

Yet the calorie count is modest: totaling 1,160 calories, well under my typical consumption. With whole plant foods, protein arrives appropriately packaged for human consumption. Think of it as nutrition in a perfect outfit.

Q: Where do you get calcium without milk?

A: Other than in clever milk commercials, once they are past calf stage, cows do *not* drink milk. So where do adult cows get the calcium they need to build those massive bones and buckets of milk? *It is abundant in the green plants they eat.* And that's where you can get your calcium, too.

Don't worry; you won't need to chew on blades of grass to beef up your bones. Plants require calcium in order to produce leaves, stems, and other solid structures. They draw this mineral directly out of the soil to package it all up nicely in a beautiful, delicious form that is easy for you to eat and absorb.

The list of dark greens that you can enjoy for getting all the calcium you need includes, for starters, romaine lettuce, chard, asparagus, kale, collard greens, broccoli, arugula, spinach, bok choy, and Brussels sprouts. A mere 1½-cup serving of kale, for example, contains 150 milligrams of calcium. Dark leafy greens also provide magnesium, an important companion to calcium. Calcium is also abundant in other plant sources such as beans.

Q: Do I need to take supplements, such as vitamins and antioxidants?

A: The vitamins and antioxidants necessary to your health—with the exception of vitamin B_{12}—are found in the colorful fruits and vegetables. Although the $500 million antioxidant supplement industry would have you believe that you can get all the antioxidant benefits you need from nutritional supplements, research favors obtaining antioxidants from real foods rather than dietary supplements. Although taking multivitamins might sound like a good idea, studies on people who take multivitamins on a regular basis reveal that supplements are not only probably ineffective, but they also can be hazardous to your health and increase disease risk.[6] The health risk may well be due to their suppressing effect of your body's own internal antioxidant mechanism—your built-in adaptive stress response that combats oxidative stress and inflammation.[7] Vitamin supplement manufacturers take one antioxidant, and concentrate it into extremely high amounts in a pill. The result is high concentrations of what could be called a pharmaceutical agent— essentially, a drug that can have unforeseen side effects.[8,9,10] The same goes for mineral supplementation, which can contribute to atherosclerotic plaque, kidney stones, and arthritis.[11,12] Have a conversation with your trusted health care provider or dietitian and do your research so that you can arrive at the best solution for your personal needs.

Q: Do you need to supplement vitamin B_{12} on a plant-based diet?

A: Yes. But does that make a diet without animal products somehow flawed? Not when you understand where the B_{12} comes from. In contrast to most vitamins, which are synthesized by plants, vitamin B_{12} is unique because it is synthesized naturally by bacteria growing in soil, water, and the intestinal tract of animals. That's why the vast majority of plants don't contain vitamin B_{12}, and any trace B_{12} in plants is due to microbial contamination from soil or manure. Modern food processing sanitizes fruits and vegetables—barring the occasional *E. coli* contamination from contact with animal products. For that reason, we can only get this particular bacteria from animal products that are . . . well, contaminated. The RDA for adults for vitamin B_{12} is 2.4 micrograms daily. Given that B_{12} absorption issues are not uncommon, 5 to 10 micrograms a day is usually recommended. See your trusted health care provider and do your research so that you can find the best solution for your personal needs.

PLANT-BASED REPLACEMENTS FOR DAIRY MILK, EGGS, AND OIL

It's fairly simple to replace animal products and oil in recipes with plant products. In many situations, the switch won't even be noticeable. As your arsenal of recipes grows, you'll find less and less need for substitutes.

DAIRY MILK REPLACEMENTS

Dairy milk is easily replaced measure for measure with plant milk. There are many nondairy milks on the market today—almond, rice, oat, soy, cashew, even hemp.

Look for plant milk brands that have the shortest list of ingredients, with no added oil. If you are aspiring to a low-fat diet, check the fat content on the label, as some plant milks are still higher in fat, such as coconut milk and some nut milks. Look for unsweetened varieties. The brand I buy most often is West Soy Unsweetened Organic. I also use almond milk and oat milk on occasion. Plant milks are easy to make inexpensively at home—recipes abound online.

When a recipe you have calls for buttermilk or sour milk, this is easily replaced as well. For each cup of buttermilk, simply take 1 cup of plant milk and add 2 teaspoons of lemon juice or vinegar. In five minutes your plant-based buttermilk will be ready.

EGG REPLACEMENTS

You'll find many plant-based cookbooks with recipes for breads, cakes, muffins, pancakes, and pies that don't call for eggs. As you voyage into new recipe territory, you can start to experiment with some of these and soon you'll find a new arsenal of egg-free favorites.

At the same time, if you want to adapt an old cherished recipe, there are multiple ways to substitute plant products for eggs. To choose the best method of replacement, without making a major project out of it, think about what role the egg plays as an ingredient in your recipe. There are two primary functions of eggs in baking: 1) as a leavening agent, for making things rise so that they are lighter and fluffier, and 2) as a binding and moistening agent, for holding things together.

Here is my short, go-to list for replacing eggs in baking, listed by the function served and best uses.

Function	To Replace One Egg	Best Use
Leavening	Dissolve 1 teaspoon baking soda in 1 tablespoon apple cider vinegar and 1 tablespoon water.	Cakes, pancakes, muffins, waffles, quick breads
Leavening	Mix 1½ teaspoons of Ener-G-Egg Replacer with 2 tablespoons water. Whisk to fully dissolve.	Cakes, pancakes, muffins, waffles, quick breads
Binding and moistening	Use ¼ cup applesauce, mashed banana, or cooked and pureed pumpkin or sweet potato.	Muffins and quick breads. Keep flavor and color in mind. Banana will add banana flavor; pumpkin will add orange color.
Binding and moistening	Stir 1 tablespoon ground golden flaxseeds or whole chia seeds in 3 tablespoons of water. Stir and let sit for about 10 minutes, or until the mixture starts to gel.	Excellent in any baked good. I use this most often. Usually I also add ½ teaspoon baking powder to the recipe's dry ingredients.

FAT AND OIL REPLACEMENTS

There are two foods I primarily use to replace oil when baking: applesauce and prune puree. I simply replace the oil with these, usually measure for measure, yet added in increments to make sure it doesn't add too much moisture. For example, if a recipe calls for ½ cup of oil or butter, I'll begin by replacing it with about ⅓ cup of applesauce, and then add more if the mixture appears to be too dry.

Mashed banana works as a replacement in similar fashion—it just seems to add more of a flavor to recipes. Sometimes that's a good thing, yet if it seems banana might overpower other flavors, stick with applesauce.

Applesauce

Applesauce is the replacement I use most often. It helps keep baked goods such as biscuits and corn bread light in color, while adding moisture and a little bit of sweetness. I buy applesauce in single-serve containers and keep them on the pantry shelf just for this purpose. Each container is about ½ cup, close to what I usually need. If the recipe only calls for ⅓ cup of oil, I'll use the full applesauce container and adjust any other moisture called for in the recipe accordingly. Alternatively, you can save by procuring larger jars of applesauce and freezing in ½-cup quantities.

Prune Puree

Prune puree, surprisingly, doesn't add a prune flavor to baked goods at all—just a nice, moist sweetness. It is best suited for use in darker-colored or spicy baked goods, such as chocolate cake and gingerbread. To make prune puree, blend ½ cup of pitted prunes and ¼ cup of water in a blender or processor until smooth. This makes about ⅔ cup. To replace 1 stick (½ cup) of butter, or ½ cup of oil, use ⅓ cup of prune puree. You can make it even easier by buying jars of prune baby food.

METRIC CONVERSION CHARTS

Measurement Guide

Abbreviation Key		
tsp	=	teaspoon
tbsp	=	tablespoon
dsp	=	dessert spoon
U.S. Standard—U.K.		
¼ tsp	=	¼ tsp (scant)
½ tsp	=	½ tsp (scant)
¾ tsp	=	½ tsp (rounded)
1 tsp	=	¾ tsp (slightly rounded)
1 tbsp	=	2 ½ tsp
¼ cup	=	¼ cup minus 1 dsp
⅓ cup	=	¼ cup plus 1 tsp
½ cup	=	⅓ cup plus 2 dsp
⅔ cup	=	½ cup plus 1 dsp
¾ cup	=	½ cup plus 2 tbsp
1 cup	=	¾ cup and 2 dsp

Oven Temperatures:

Fahrenheit (F)—Celcius (C)

250°F	=	120°C
275°F	=	140°C
300°F	=	150°C
325°F	=	160°C
350°F	=	180°C
375°F	=	190°C
400°F	=	200°C
425°F	=	220°C
450°F	=	230°C
475°F	=	245°C
500°F	=	260°C

ENDNOTES

Chapter 1

1. Nick Cooney, *Veganomics* (New York: Lantern Press, 2014).
2. Bill Gates, "The Future of Food," *The Gates Notes*, March 21, 2013, www.gatesnotes.com/About-Bill-Gates/Future-of-Food-Michael-Pollan-Q-and-A.
3. U.S. Department of Agriculture, "Food Consumption and Nutrient Intakes," USDA Economic Research Service, 2009, www.ers.usda.gov/data-products/food-consumption-and-nutrient-intakes.aspx#.Uzb6aPldWSo.
4. New York Coalition for Health School Food, "US Food Consumption as Percent of Calories," www.healthyschoolfood.org/nutrition101.htm.
5. F. B. Hu and W. C. Willett, "Optimal Diets for Prevention of Coronary Heart Disease," *JAMA* 288, no. 20 (November 27, 2002): 2569–78.
6. F. B. Hu, "Plant-based foods and prevention of cardiovascular disease: an overview," *American Journal of Clinical Nutrition* 78 (2003): 544S–51S.
7. D. L. Hoyert and J. Q. Xu, "Deaths: Preliminary data for 2011," *National Vital Statistics Reports* 61 (2012).
8. K. L. Tucker, J. Hallfrisch, N. Qiao, et al., "The Combination of High Fruit and Vegetable and Low Saturated Fat Intakes Is More Protective Against Mortality in Aging Men Than Is Either Alone: The Baltimore Longitudinal Study of Aging," *Journal of Nutrition* 135 (2005): 556–61.
9. D. Ornish, S. E. Brown, L. W. Scherwitz, et al., "Can Lifestyle Changes Reverse Coronary Heart Disease? The Lifestyle Heart Trial," *The Lancet* 336, no. 8708 (July 21, 1990): 129–33.
10. D. Ornish, L. W. Scherwitz, et al., "Intensive Lifestyle Changes for Reversal of Coronary Heart Disease," *JAMA* 280, no. 23 (December 16, 1998): 2001–7.
11. Caldwell B. Esselstyn, *Prevent and Reverse Heart Disease* (New York: Penguin Group, 2007).
12. Preventative Medicine Research Institute, "Ornish Programs Reimbursed by Medicare," www.pmri.org/certified_programs.html.
13. Phillip J. Tuso, Mohamed H. Ismail, Benjamin P. Ha, and Carole Bartolotto, "Nutritional Update for Physicians: Plant-Based Diets," *Permanente Journal* 17, no. 2 (Spring 2013): 61–66.
14. Union of Concerned Scientists, "Investing in Healthy Food Will Save Lives and Dollars," www.ucsusa.org/food_and_agriculture/solutions/expand-healthy-food-access/11-trillion-reward.html.
15. Hongyu Wu, Alan J. Flint, Frank B. Hu, et al., "Association Between Dietary Whole Grain Intake and Risk of Mortality," *JAMA Internal Medicine*, January 5, 2015 (online).
16. Academy of Nutrition and Dietetics, "The Basics of the Nutrition Facts Panel," http://www.eatright.org/resource/food/nutrition/nutrition-facts-and-food-labels/the-basics-of-the-nutrition-facts-panel (accessed February 2014).
17. USDA, "Healthy Eating Tips," www.choosemyplate.gov/healthy-eating-tips/tips-for-vegetarian.html.
18. Scott Cooney, "Are We Eating Too Much Protein?" *Eat Drink Better*, http://eatdrinkbetter.com/2014/10/22/are-we-eating-too-much-protein.
19. T. Colin Campbell, "The Mystique of Protein and Its Implications," Center for Nutrition Studies, http://nutritionstudies.org/mystique-of-protein-implications (accessed January 19, 2014).

20. T. Colin Campbell, PhD, has received more than seventy grant years of peer-reviewed research funding, much of which was funded by the U.S. National Institutes of Health (NIH), and has authored more than 300 research papers. His work is regarded by many as the definitive epidemiological examination of the relationship between diet and disease.

21. N. E. Allen, P. N Appleby, et al., "The Associations of Diet with Serum Insulin-Like Growth Factor I and Its Main Binding Proteins in 292 Women Meat-Eaters, Vegetarians, and Vegans," *Cancer Epidemiology, Biomarkers and Prevention* 11, no. 11 (2002): 1441–48.

22. M. Rincon, E. Rudin, and N. Barzilai, "The Insulin/IGF-1 Signaling in Mammals and Its Relevance to Human Longevity," *Experimental Gerontology* 40, no. 11 (2005): 873–77.

23. Andrew G. Renehan et al., "Insulin-Like Growth Factor (IGF)-I, IGF Binding Protein-3, and Cancer Risk: Systematic Review and Meta-Regression Analysis," *The Lancet* 363 (2014): 1346–53.

24. Luigi Fontana, Samuel Klein, and John O Holloszy, "Long-Term Low-Protein, Low-Calorie Diet and Endurance Exercise Modulate Metabolic Factors Associated with Cancer Risk," *American Journal of Clinical Nutrition* 84 (2006): 1456–62.

25. S. J. Moschos and C. S. Mantzoros, "The Role of the IGF System in Cancer: From Basic to Clinical Studies and Clinical Applications," *Oncology* 63, no. 4 (2002): 317–32.

26. M. M. Chitnis, J. S. Yuen, et al., "The Type 1 Insulin-Like Growth Factor Receptor Pathway," *Clinical Cancer Research* 14 (2008): 6364–70.

27. H. Werner and I. Bruchim, "The Insulin-Like Growth Factor-I Receptor as an Oncogene," *Archives of Physiology and Biochemistry* 115, no. 2 (June 2009): 58–71.

28. M. S. Sandhu, D. B. Dunger, and E. L. Giovannucci, "Insulin, Insulin-Like Growth Factor-I (IGF-I), IGF Binding Proteins, Their Biologic Interactions, and Colorectal Cancer," *Journal of the National Cancer Institute* 94 (2002): 972–80.

29. T. Colin Campbell, "The Protein Juggernaut Has Deep Roots," *Forks Over Knives*, www.forksoverknives.com/the-protein-juggernaut-has-deep-roots (accessed October 15, 2013).

30. "Would We Be Healthier with a Vegan Diet?" *Wall Street Journal*, September 18, 2012, www.wsj.com/articles/SB10000872396390444184704577587174077811182.

31. T. Colin Campbell and Thomas M. Campbell, *The China Study* (Dallas: BenBella Books, 2005).

32. V. R. Young and P. L. Pellett, "Plant Proteins in Relation to Human Protein and Amino Acid Nutrition," *American Journal of Clinical Nutrition* 59, no. (1994): 1203S–12S.

33. C. Esselstyn and M. Golubic, "The Nutritional Reversal of Cardiovascular Disease: Fact or Fiction? Three Cases," *Experimental & Clinical Cardiology* 20, no. 7 (2014): 1901–8.

34. Expert panel, "Food, Nutrition, Physical Activity, and the Prevention of Cancer, a Global Perspective," American Institute for Cancer Research/World Cancer Research Fund, 1997, www.dietandcancerreport.org/cancer_resource_center/downloads/summary/english.pdf.

35. N. D. Barnard, A. E. Bunner, U. Agarwal. "Saturated and Trans Fats and Dementia: A Systematic Review," *Neurobiology of Aging* 35 (2014): S65–S73.

36. T. Colin Campbell and Howard Jacobson, *Whole: Rethinking the Science of Nutrition* (Dallas: BenBella Books, 2013).

37. An Pan et al., "Red Meat Consumption and Mortality," *Archives of Internal Medicine* 172 (2012): 555–63.

38. Harvard School of Public Health, "Red Meat Consumption Linked to Increased Risk of Total, Cardiovascular, and Cancer Mortality," March 12, 2012, www.hsph.harvard.edu/news/press-releases/red-meat-consumption-linked-to-increased-risk-of-total-cardiovascular-and-cancer-mortality.

39. "Cholesterol Count of Foods," UCSF Medical Center, www.ucsfhealth.org/education/ cholesterol_content_of_foods.

40. Neal Barnard, "Editorial: The Chicken Myth," *Good Medicine* XV, no. 3 (Summer 2006), Physicians Committee for Responsible Medicine, www.pcrm.org/good-medicine/2006/ summer/editorial-the-chicken-myth.

41. Neal Barnard, "Fecal Contamination in Retail Chicken Products," A Report from the Physicians Committee for Responsible Medicine, April 2012, www.pcrm.org/health/ reports/fecal-contamination-in-retail-chicken-products.

42. Jennifer Reilly, "Grilled Chicken Contains Cancer-Causing Compounds," *Good Medicine* XV, no. 3 (Summer 2006), Physicians Committee for Responsible Medicine, www.pcrm.org/ good-medicine/2006/summer/playing-with-fire-grilled-chicken-contains-cancer.

43. Y. Li, C. Zhou, X. Zhou, and L. Li, "Egg Consumption and Risk of Cardiovascular Diseases and Diabetes: A Meta-Analysis," *Atherosclerosis* 229, no. 2 (April 2013): 524–30.

44. E. L. Richman, S. A. Kenfield, M. J. Stampfer, E. L. Giovannucci, and J. M. Chan, "Egg, Red Meat, and Poultry Intake and Risk of Lethal Prostate Cancer in the Prostate Specific Antigen-Era: Incidence and Survival," *Cancer Prevention Research* 4, no. 12 (December 2011): 2110–21.

45. John McDougall, "Dairy Products and 10 False Promises," *The McDougall Newsletter*, April 2003, www.nealhendrickson.com/mcdougall/030400pudairyproductsfalsepromises.htm.

46. T. Saukkonen, S. M. Virtanen, M. Karppinen, et al., "Significance of Cow's Milk Protein Antibodies as Risk Factor for Childhood IDDM: Interaction with Dietary Cow's Milk Intake and HLA-DQB1 Genotype," *Dibetologia* 41, no. 1 (January 1998): 72–78.

47. Joseph Keon, *Whitewash: The Disturbing Truth About Cow's Milk and Your Health* (Gabriola Island, BC: New Society Publishers, 2010).

48. Amy Lanou and Michael Castleman, *Building Bone Vitality* (New York: McGraw Hill, 2009).

49. K. Michaëlsson, A. Wolk, S. Langenskiöld, et al., "Milk Intake and Risk of Mortality and Fractures in Women and Men: Cohort Studies," *BMJ* 349 (2014): g6015.

50. A. J. Lanour, "Should Dairy Be Recommended as Part of a Healthy Vegetarian Diet? Counterpoint," *American Journal of Clinical Nutrition* 89, no. 5 (May 2009): 1638S–42S.

51. L. A. Frassetto, "Worldwide Incidence of Hip Fracture in Elderly Women: Relation to Consumption of Animal and Vegetable Foods," *Journal of Gerontology*: Series A 55, no. 10 (October 5, 2000): 585–92.

52. Rocket fuel—perchlorate—can affect the thyroid gland's ability to make essential hormones, interfering with normal brain development and growth. For fetuses, infants, and children, such disruption can cause lowered IQ, mental retardation, loss of hearing and speech, and motor skill deficits.

53. Environmental Working Group, "Rocket Fuel in Cows' Milk—Perchlorate," June 22, 2004, www.ewg.org/research/rocket-fuel-cows-milk-perchlorate.

54. Detected in breast milk, dairy milk, produce, and many other foods and plants, perchlorate has leaked from military bases and defense and aerospace contractors' plants in at least twenty-two states, contaminating drinking water for millions of Americans.

55. Environmental Working Group, "EPA: Rocket Fuel Contaminant Safe for Nation's Drinking Water," October 3, 2008, www.ewg.org/news/news-releases/2008/10/03/epa-rocket-fuel -contaminant-safe-nation%E2%80%99s-drinking-water.

56. P. C. B. Vianna, G. Mazal, et al., "Microbial and Sensory Changes Throughout the Ripening of Prato Cheese Made from Milk with Different Levels of Somatic Cells," *Journal of Dairy Science* 91, no. 5 (May 2008): 1743–50.

57. Joseph Keon, *Whitewash: The Disbturbing Truth About Cow's Milk and Your Health*. (New Society Publishers, 2010).

58. Kathy Freston, "A Cure for Cancer? Eating a Plant-Based Diet," *The Huffington Post*, September 24, 2009, www.huffingtonpost.com/kathy-freston/a-cure-for-cancer-eating_b_298282.html.

59. David Robinson Simon, *Meatonomics* (San Francisco: Conari Press, 2013).

60. Carrie Hibar, "Understanding Concentrated Animal Feeding Operations and Their Impact on Communities," National Association of Local Boards of Health, 2010, www.cdc.gov/nceh/ehs/docs/understanding_cafos_nalboh.pdf.

61. Robert A. Kanaly et al., "Energy Flow, Environment and Ethical Implications for Meat Production," UNESCO Bangkok, 2010, http://unesdoc.unesco.org/images/0018/001897/189774e.pdf.

62. Bill Gates, "Food Is Ripe for Innovation," March 21, 2013, http://mashable.com/2013/03/21/bill-gates-future-of-food.

63. V. R. Young and P. L. Pellett, "Plant Proteins in Relation to Human Protein and Amino Acid Nutrition," *American Journal of Clinical Nutrition* 59 (May 1994): 1203S–12S.

64. Richard Oppenlander, *Food Choice and Sustainability* (Minneapolis: Langdon Street Press, 2013).

65. "Some Dangers of Hormones in Milk," *Rachel's Hazardous Waste News* No. 382, Environmental Research Foundation, March 1994, www.ejnet.org/rachel/rhwn382.htm.

66. Robert M. Kradjian, "The Milk Letter: A Message to My Patients," www.notmilk.com/kradjian.html.

67. I. R. Dohoo, L. DesCôteaux, K. Leslie, et al., "A Meta-Analysis Review of the Effects of Recombinant Bovine Somatotropin: 2. Effects on Animal Health, Reproductive Performance, and Culling," *Canadian Journal of Veterinary Research* 67, no. 4 (2003): 252–64.

68. "Cows on Factory Farms," ASPCA, www.aspca.org/fight-cruelty/farm-animal-cruelty/cows-factory-farms.

69. Roberto A. Ferdman, "The Not-So-Humane Way 'Humanely Raised' Chickens Are Being Raised," *Washington Post*, December 8, 2014, www.washingtonpost.com/blogs/wonkblog/wp/2014/12/08/the-not-so-humane-way-humanely-raised-chickens-are-being-raised.

70. Bruce Friedrich, "The Cruelest of All Factory Farm Products: Eggs from Caged Hens," *The Huffington Post*, January 14, 2013, www.huffingtonpost.com/bruce-friedrich/eggs-from-caged-hens_b_2458525.html.

71. Gidon Eshel, interview by Ira Platow, "What's the Real Cost of Your Steak?" *Science Friday*, NPR, July 25, 2013, http://sciencefriday.com/segment/07/25/2014/what-s-the-real-cost-of-your-steak.html.

72. James McWilliams, "Small, Free-Range Egg Producers Can't Escape Problems of Factory Farms," *Forbes*, October 23, 2013, www.forbes.com/sites/jamesmcwilliams/2013/10/23/small-free-range-egg-producers-cant-escape-problems-of-factory-farms.

73. Howard Lyman, *Mad Cowboy* (New York: Scribner, 2001).

74. Richard Oppenlander, *Food Choice and Sustainability* (Minneapolis: Langdon Street Press, 2013).

75. R. P. Friedland, R. B. Peterson, and R. Rubenstein, "Bovine Spongiform Encephalopathy and Aquaculture," *Journal of Alzheimer's Disease* 17 (2009): 277–79.

76. Richard Oppenlander, *Food Choice and Sustainability* (Minneapolis: Langdon Street Press, 2013).

77. Evelyn Theiss, "Should the USDA Make Dietary Guidelines While It Promotes Meat and Dairy Industry?" *Cleveland Plain Dealer*, March 7, 2011.

78. Patrick A. Malone, "New Dietary Guidelines May Be Overtly Influenced by Agribusiness," *DC Medical Malpractice and Patient Safety Blog*, February 19, 2011, www.protectpatientsblog.com/2011/02/new_dietary_guidelines_may_be.html.

79. Theiss, "Should the USDA Make Dietary Guidelines?"

80. "Calcium and Milk: What's Best for Your Bones and Health?" Harvard School of Public Health, www.hsph.harvard.edu/nutritionsource/what-should-you-eat/calcium-and-milk.

81. "New U.S. Dietary Guidelines: Progress, Not Perfection," Harvard School of Public Health, www.hsph.harvard.edu/nutritionsource/dietary-guidelines-2010.

82. Richard Volpe and Abigail Okrent, "Assessing the Healthfulness of Consumers' Grocery Purchases," *Economic Information Bulletin*, no. 102, November 2012.

83. David R. Jacobs et al., "Food, Plant Food, and Vegetarian Diets in the US Dietary Guidelines: Conclusions of an Expert Panel," *American Journal of Clinical Nutrition* 89, no. 5 (May 2009): 1549S–52S.

84. 2015 Dietary Guidelines Advisory Committee Meeting 3, Sponsored by the U.S. Department of Health and Human Services (HHS) U.S. Department of Agriculture (USDA), March 14, 2014, www.health.gov/dietaryguidelines/DGAC-Meeting-3-Summary-508.pdf.

85. Eliza Barclay, "James Cameron-Backed School to Terminate Meat and Dairy," NPR, June 8, 2014, http://www.npr.org/blogs/thesalt/2014/06/08/305860073/james-cameron-backed-school-to-terminate-meat-and-dairy.

86. Suzy Amis Cameron, in discussion with the author, November 10, 2014.

87. Ryan Mac, "Bill Gates–Backed Food Startup Hampton Creek Begins to Come Out of Shell, Make Money," *Forbes*, May 13, 2014, www.forbes.com/sites/ryanmac/2014/05/13/bill-gates-backed-food-startup-hampton-creek-begins-to-come-out-of-shell-make-money.

88. Stephanie M. Lee, "Hampton Creek Takes Crack at Breaking Up Egg Industry," *SFGate*, August 16, 2014, www.sfgate.com/food/article/Hampton-Creek-takes-crack-at-breaking-up-egg-5693576.php#page-1.

Chapter 2

1. Neal Barnard, *Breaking the Food Seduction* (New York: St. Martin's Press, 2003).

2. Anna Schecter and Drew Sandholm, "Dehorning: 'Standard Practice' on Dairy Farms," ABC News, January 28, 2010, http://abcnews.go.com/Blotter/dehorning-standard-practice-dairy-farms/story?id=9658414.

Chapter 3

1. Phillip J. Tuso, Mohamed H. Ismail, Benjamin P. Ha, and Carole Bartolotto, "Nutritional Update for Physicians: Plant-Based Diets" *Permanente Journal* 17, no. 2 (Spring 2013): 61–66.

2. The "three food categories" is a brilliant perspective I learned in an interview with Dr. T. Colin Campbell while preparing the manuscript for this book.

3. G. H. Perry, N. J. Dominy, K. G. Claw, A. S. Lee, et al., "Diet and the Evolution of Human Amylase Gene Copy Number Variation," *Nature Genetics* 39 (2007): 1256–60.

4. Carbophobia, according to S. N. Cheuvront, PhD, RD, in a 2003 *American Journal of Clinical Nutrition* review of low-carb diets and theories, is "a form of nutrition misinformation infused into the American psyche through multiple advertising avenues that include magazine ads, television infomercials and especially best selling diet books."

5. "Pringles Are Not 'Potato Crisps,'" BBC News, July 4, 2008, http://news.bbc.co.uk/2/hi/business/7490346.stm.

6. N. P. Hays and S. B. Roberts, "Aspects of Eating Behaviors 'Disinhibition' and 'Restraint' Are Related to Weight Gain and BMI in Women," *Obesity* 16, no. 1 (2008): 52–58.

Chapter 4

1. K. W. Heaton, S. N. Marcus, P. M. Emmett, and C. H. Bolton, "Particle Size of Wheat, Maize, and Oat Test Meals: Effects on Plasma Glucose and Insulin Responses and on the Rate of Starch Digestion in Vitro," *American Journal of Clinical Nutrition* 47, no. 4 (April 1988): 675–82.

2. S. H. Holt and J. B. Miller, "Particle Size, Satiety and the Glycaemic Response," *European Journal of Clinical Nutrition* 48, no. 7 (July 1994): 496–502.

3. Elizabeth A. Bell, V. H. Castellanos, C. L. Pelkman, M. L. Thorwart, and B. J. Rolls, "Energy Density of Foods Affects Energy Intake in Normal-Weight Women," *American Journal of Clinical Nutrition* 67 (1998): 412–20.

4. Pamela Popper, *Dr. Pam Popper's Health News You Can Use* 8, no. 26 (June 28, 2010), www.wellnessforum.com/Messager/Newsletters/1277743472656.html.

5. K. A. Houpt, "Gastrointestinal Factors in Hunger and Satiety," *Neuroscience & Biobehavioral Reviews* 6, no. 2 (Summer 1982): 145–64.

6. J. A. Deutsch, "The Role of the Stomach in Eating," *American Journal of Clinical Nutrition* 42, Suppl. no. 5 (November 1985): 1040–43.

7. M. J. Clark and J. L. Slavin, "The Effect of Fiber on Satiety and Food Intake: A Systematic Review," *Journal of the American College of Nutrition* 32 (2013): 200–11.

8. L. Brown, B. Rosner, W. W. Willett, and F. M. Sacks, "Cholesterol-Lowering Effects of Dietary Fiber: A Meta-Analysis," *American Journal of Clinical Nutrition* 69, no. 1 (January 1999): 30–42.

9. J. Montonen, P. Knekt, R. Järvinen, A. Aromaa, and A. Reunanen, "Whole-Grain and Fiber Intake and the Incidence of Type 2 Diabetes," *American Journal of Clinical Nutrition* 77, no. 3 (2003): 622–29.

10. USDA, "Dietary Guidelines for Americans," www.cnpp.usda.gov/Publications/DietaryGuidelines/2010/PolicyDoc/Chapter4.pdf.

11. S. Liu, "Whole-Grain Foods, Dietary Fiber, and Type 2 Diabetes: Searching for a Kernel of Truth," *American Journal of Clinical Nutrition* 77, no. 3 (March 2003): 527–29.

12. S. Dayton, S. Hashimoto, W. Dixon, and M. L. Pearce, "Composition of Lipids in Human Serum and Adipose Tissue During Prolonged Feeding of a Diet High in Unsaturated Fat," *Journal of Lipid Research* 7, no. 1 (January 1966): 103–11.

13. Tracy J. Horton, Holly Drougas, Amy Brachey, George W. Reed, John C. Peters, and James O. Hill, "Fat and Carbohydrate Overfeeding in Humans: Different Effects on Energy Storage," *American Journal of Clinical Nutrition* 62, no. 1 (July 1995): 19–29.

14. S. H. Holt, H. J. Delargy, C. L. Lawton, and J. E. Blundell, "The Effects of High-Carbohydrate vs High-Fat Breakfasts on Feelings of Fullness and Alertness, and Subsequent Food Intake," *International Journal of Food Sciences and Nutrition* 50, no. 1 (January 1999): 13–28.

15. R. J. Stubbs, C. G. Harbron, P. R. Murgatroyd, and A. M. Prentice, "Covert Manipulation of Dietary Fat to Carbohydrate and Energy Density: Effect on Substrate Flux and Food Intake in Men Eating Ad Libitum," *American Journal of Clinical Nutrition* 62, no. 2 (1995): 316–29.

16. S. D. Poppitt and A. M. Prentice, "Energy Density and Its Role in the Control of Food Intake: Evidence from Metabolic and Community Studies," *Appetite* 26, no. 2 (April 1996): 153–74.

17. B. J. Rolls, S. Kim-Harris, M. W. Fischman, R. W. Foltin, T. H. Moran, and S. A. Stoner, "Satiety After Preloads with Different Amounts of Fat and Carbohydrate: Implications for Obesity," *American Journal of Clinical Nutrition* 60, no. 4 (October 1994): 476–78.

18. C. L. Lawton, V. J. Burley, J. K. Wales, and J. E. Blundell, "Dietary Fat and Appetite Control in Obese Subjects: Weak Effects on Satiation and Satiety," *International Journal of Obesity* 17 (1993): 409–16.

19. J. R. Cotton, V. J. Burley, J. A. Westrate, and J. E. Blundell, "Dietary Fat and Appetite: Similarities and Differences in the Satiating Effect of Meals Supplemented with Fat or Carbohydrate," *Journal of Human Nutrition and Dietetics* 7 (1994): 11–24.

20. S. M. Green et al., "Effect of Fat- and Sucrose-Containing Foods on the Size of Eating Episodes and Energy Intake in Lean Males: Potential for Causing Overconsumption," *European Journal of Clinical Nutrition* 48, no. 8 (1994): 547–55.

21. S. M. Green and J. E. Blundell, "Effect of Fat- and Sucrose- Containing Foods on the Size of Eating Episodes and Energy Intake in Lean Dietary Restrained and Unrestrained Females: Potential for Causing Overconsumption," *European Journal of Clinical Nutrition* 50, no. 9 (1996): 625–35.

22. Neal Barnard, *Turn Off the Fat Genes* (New York: Harmony Books, 2001).

23. Gina Kolata, "Mediterranean Diet Shown to Ward Off Heart Attack and Stroke," *New York Times*, February 25, 2013, www.nytimes.com/2013/02/26/health/mediterranean-diet-can-cut-heart-disease-study-finds.html?pagewanted=all&_r=0.

24. Ramón Estruch et al., "Primary Prevention of Cardiovascular Disease with a Mediterranean Diet," *New England Journal of Medicine* 368 (April 4, 2013): 1279–90.

25. D. H. Blankenhorn, R. L. Johnson, W. J. Mack, et al., "The Influence of Diet on the Appearance of New Lesions in Human Coronary Arteries," *JAMA* 263, no. 12 (March 23–30, 1990): 1646–52.

26. R. A. Vogel, M. C. Corretti, and G. D. Plotnick, "The Postprandial Effect of Components of the Mediterranean Diet on Endothelial Function," *Journal of the American College of Cardiology* 36, no. 5 (November 1, 2000): 1455–60.

27. Julieanna Hever, *The Vegiterranean Diet* (Boston: Da Capo Press, 2014).

28. Gabrielle M. Turner-McGrievy, Charis R. Davidson, Ellen E. Wingard, Sara Wilcox, and Edward A. Frongillo, "Comparative Effectiveness of Plant-Based Diets for Weight Loss: A Randomized Controlled Trial of Five Different Diets," *Nutrition* 31, no. 2 (2014): 350–58.

29. "Vegan Diet Best for Weight Loss Even with Carbohydrate Consumption, Study Finds," *Science Daily*, November 6, 2014, www.sciencedaily.com/releases/2014/11/141106101732.htm.

30. N. D. Barnard, S. M. Levin, and Y. Yokoyama, "A Systematic Review and Meta-Analysis of Changes in Body Weight in Clinical Trials of Vegetarian Diets," *Journal of the Academy of Nutrition and Dietetics*, published online January 17, 2015.

31. T. Colin Campbell and Junshi Chen, "Energy Balance: Interpretation of Data from Rural China," *Toxicological Sciences* 52 (Supplement) (1999): 87–94.

32. D. S. Miller and P. B. Payne, "Weight Maintenance and Food Intake," *Journal of Nutrition* 78, no. 3 (November 1, 1962): 255–62.

33. Tracy J. Horton, Holly Drougas, Amy Brachey, George W. Reed, John C. Peters, and James O. Hill, "Fat and Carbohydrate Overfeeding in Humans: Different Effects on Energy Storage," *American Journal of Clinical Nutrition* 62, no. 1 (July 1995): 19–29.

34. Vincent P. Dole, Irving L. Schwartz, Thaysen Hess, Niels A. Thorn, and Lawrence Silver, "Treatment of Obesity with a Low Protein Calorically Unrestricted Diet," *American Journal of Clinical Nutrition* 2, no. 6 (November 1954): 381–91.

Chapter 5

1. Norman J. Temple and Joy Fraser, "Food Labels: A Critical Assessment," *Nutrition Journal* 30, no. 3 (March 2013): 257–60.
2. U.S. FDA, "How to Understand and Use the Nutrition Facts Label," www.fda.gov/Food/IngredientsPackagingLabeling/LabelingNutrition/ucm274593.htm.
3. G. Cowburn and L. Stockley, "Consumer Understanding and Use of Nutrition Labelling: A Systematic Review," *Public Health Nutrition* 8, no. 1 (February 2005): 21–28.
4. Temple, "Food Labels," 258.
5. Caroline Scott-Thomas, "European Trade Organisations 'Deeply Concerned' by UK Traffic Light Labeling," June 21, 2013, www.foodnavigator.com/Legislation/European-trade-organisations-deeply-concerned-by-UK-traffic-light-labelling/?utm_source=newsletter_daily&utm_medium=email&utm_campaign=Newsletter%2BDaily&c=bdxIOU1sHYoqXBDFMxXC9Q%3D%3D.
6. "Why Food 'Traffic-Light' Labels Did Not Happen," BBC News Health, July 11, 2012, www.bbc.com/news/health-18767425.

Chapter 6

1. Caldwell Esselstyn, personal interview, December 11, 2014.
2. Caldwell Esselstyn and Mladen Golubic, "The Nutritional Reversal of Cardiovascular Disease—Fact or Fiction? Three Case Reports," *Experimental & Clinical Cardiology* 20, no. 7 (2014): 1901–8.

Chapter 7

1. USDA Center for Nutrition Policy and Promotion, "Dietary Guidelines for Americans," 2010, www.cnpp.usda.gov/DietaryGuidelines.
2. M. McCrory, B. Hamaker, J. Lovejoy, and P. Eichelsdoerfer, "Pulse Consumption, Satiety, and Weight Management," *Advances in Nutrition* 1 (November 2010): 17–30.
3. R. C. Mollard, C. L. Wong, B. L. Luhovyy, and G. H. Anderson, "First and Second Meal Effects of Pulses on Blood Glucose, Appetite, and Food Intake at a Later Meal," *Applied Physiology, Nutrition, and Metabolism* 36, no. 5 (October 2011): 634–42.
4. Joanne Slavin and Angela Bonnema, "The 'Second Meal' Effect of Dry Beans and Lentils Offers Health Benefits," http://beaninstitute.com/the-second-meal-effect-of-dry-beans-and-lentils-offers-health-benefits/#sthash.WdI5IJny.dpuf.
5. B. J. Rolls, L. S. Roe, J. S. Meengs, "Salad and Satiety: Energy Density and Portion Size of a First-Course Salad Affect Energy Intake at Lunch," *Journal of the American Dietetic Association* 104, no. 10 (October 2004): 1570–76.
6. Julie E. Flood and Barbara J. Rolls, "Soup Preloads in a Variety of Forms Reduce Meal Energy Intake," *Appetite* 49, no. 3 (November 2007): 626–34.

Chapter 8

1. Carla R. McGill et al., "Consumption of Purple/Blue Produce Is Associated with Increased Nutrient Intake and Reduced Risk for Metabolic Syndrome," *American Journal of Lifestyle Medicine* 5, no. 3 (2011): 279–90.

Chapter 10

1. Solveig A. Cunningham, Michael R. Kramer, and K. M. Venkat Narayan, "Incidence of Childhood Obesity in the United States," *New England Journal of Medicine* 370 (January 30, 2014): 403–11.

2. Philip J. Tuso et al., "Nutritional Update for Physicians: Plant-Based Diets," *Permanente Journal* 17 (2013): 61–66.

3. David R. Just and Brian Wansink, "Smarter Lunchrooms: Using Behavioral Economics to Improve Meal Selection," *Choices Magazine*, www.choicesmagazine.org/magazine/article.php?article=87.

4. Ibid.

5. "Children Eat More Vegetables When Allowed to Choose," Canal UGR, May 30, 2011, http://canalugr.es/social-economic-and-legal-sciences/item/50039.

6. Kay Sheppard, "The Science of Refined Food Addiction," *Counselor Magazine*, September 28, 2009, http://kaysheppard.com/articles/refined-food-addiction.

7. Nicole M. Avena, Pedro Rada, and Bartley G. Hoebel, "Evidence for Sugar Addiction: Behavioral and Neurochemical Effects of Intermittent, Excessive Sugar Intake," *Neuroscience & Biobehavioral Reviews* 32, no. 1 (2008): 20–39.

8. Neal Barnard, *Breaking the Food Seduction: The Hidden Reasons Behind Food Cravings* (New York: St. Martin's Press, 2003).

9. S. H. Ahmed, K. Guillem, and Y. Vandaele, "Sugar Addiction: Pushing the Drug-Sugar Analogy to the Limit," *Current Opinion in Clinical Nutrition and Metabolic Care* 16, no. 4 (July 2013): 434–39.

10. James DiNicolantonio, "Is Sugar More Addictive Than Cocaine?" *Here and Now*, NPR, January 7, 2015, https://hereandnow.wbur.org/2015/01/07/sugar-health-research.

11. David A. Kessler, *The End of Overeating. Taking Control of the Insatiable American Appetite* (New York: Rodale Books, 2009).

12. J. P. Pinel, S. Assanand, and D. R. Lehman, "Hunger, Eating and Ill Health," *American Psychologist* 55, no. 10 (2000): 1105–16.

Chapter 11

1. P. Feng, L. Huang, and H. Wang Chem, "Taste Bud Homeostasis in Health, Disease, and Aging," *Chemical Senses* 39, no. 1 (January 2014): 3–16.

2. John McDougall, "Eat Yourself Impotent," *The McDougall Newsletter*, May 2008, www.drmcdougall.com/misc/2008nl/may/fav5.htm.

Chapter 12

1. Ana C. Pereira, Dan E. Huddleston, Adam M. Brickman, et al., "An in Vivo Correlate of Exercise-Induced Neurogenesis in the Adult Dentate Gyrus," *Proceedings of the National Academy of Sciences* 104, no. 13 (2007): 5638–43.

2.   A. R. Ozburn, R. A. Harris, and Y. A. Blednov, "Wheel Running, Voluntary Ethanol Consumption, and Hedonic Substitution," *Alcohol* 42 (August 2008): 417–24.

3.   S. Brené, A. Bjørnebekk, E. Åberg, A. A. Mathé, L. Olson, and M. Werme, "Running Is Rewarding and Antidepressive," *Physiology & Behavior* 92, nos. 1–2 (September 10, 2007): 136–40.

4.   John Ratey, *Spark: The Revolutionary New Science of Exercise and the Brain* (New York: Little, Brown and Company, 2008).

5.   R. E. Andersen, T. A. Wadden, S. J. Bartlett, B. Zemel, T. J. Verde, and S. C. Franckowiak, "Effects of Lifestyle Activity vs Structured Aerobic Exercise in Obese Women: A Randomized Trial," *JAMA* 281, no. 4 (January 27, 1999): 335–40.

6.   J. A. Zoladz and A. J. Pilc, "The Effect of Physical Activity on the Brain Derived Neurotrophic Factor: From Animal to Human Studies," *Journal of Physiology and Pharmacology* 61, no. 5 (October 2010): 533–41.

7.   K. Hötting and B. Röder, "Beneficial Effects of Physical Exercise on Neuroplasticity and Cognition," *Neuroscience & Biobehavioral Reviews* 37, no. 9 Pt. B (November 2013): 2243–57.

8.   John Ratey, *Spark: The Revolutionary New Science of Exercise and the Brain* (New York: Little, Brown and Company, 2008).

9.   K. Hötting and B. Röder, "Beneficial Effects of Physical Exercise on Neuroplasticity and Cognition," *Neuroscience & Biobehavioral Reviews* 37, no. 9 Pt. B (November 2013): 2243–57.

10.   P. T. Katzmarzyk, "Physical Activity, Sedentary Behavior, and Health: Paradigm Paralysis or Paradigm Shift?" *Diabetes* 59, no. 11 (November 2010): 2717–25.

11.   Neville Owen et al., "Too Much Sitting: The Population-Health Science of Sedentary Behavior," *Exercise and Sport Sciences Reviews* 38, no. 3 (2010): 105–13.

12.   L. Kravitz, "Too Much Sitting Is Hazardous to Your Health," *Idea Fitness Journal* 6, no. 9 (October 2009): 14–17.

13.   Adapted from ibid.

14.   Lani Muelrath, *Fit Quickies: 5-Minute Targeted Body-Shaping Workouts* (New York: Alpha Group Penguin Publishing, 2013).

15.   G. N. Healy, D. W. Dunstan, J. Salmon, et al., "Breaks in Sedentary Time: Beneficial Associations with Metabolic Risk," *Diabetes Care* 31 (2008): 661–66.

16.   C. E. Garber et al., "Quantity and Quality of Exercise for Developing and Maintaining Cardiorespiratory, Musculoskeletal, and Neuromotor Fitness in Apparently Healthy Adults: Guidance for Prescribing Exercise," *Medicine & Science in Sports & Exercise* 43, no. 7 (2011): 1334–59.

17.   "Weight Control and Diet," University of Maryland Medical Center, http://umm.edu/health/medical/reports/articles/weight-control-and-diet.

18.   M. Fumoto et al., "Ventral Prefrontal Cortex and Serotonergic System Activation During Pedaling Exercise Induces Negative Mood Improvement and Increased Alpha Band in EEG," *Behavioural Brain Research* 213, no. 1 (November 12, 2010): 1–9.

19.   M. H. Murphy and A. E. Hardman, "Training Effects of Short and Long Bouts of Brisk Walking in Sedentary Women," *Medicine & Science in Sports & Exercise* 30, no. 1 (January 1998): 152–57.

20.   D. R. Crabtree et al., "The Effects of High-Intensity Exercise on Neural Responses to Images of Food," *American Journal of Clinical Nutrition* 99, no. 2 (February 2014): 258–67.

21. John Ratey, *Spark: The Revolutionary New Science of Exercise and the Brain* (New York: Little, Brown and Company, 2008).

22. P. J. O'Connor, M. P. Herring, and A. Caravalho, "Mental Health Benefits of Strength Training in Adults," *American Journal of Lifestyle Medicine* 4, no. 5 (2010): 377–96.

23. T. Tsutsumi, B. M. Don, L. D. Zaichkowsky, and L. L. Delizonna, "Physical Fitness and Psychological Benefits of Strength Training in Community Dwelling Older Adults," *Applied Human Science Journal of Physiological Anthropology* 16, no. 6 (November 1997): 257–66.

24. S. G. Trost, N. Owen, A. E. Bauman, J. F. Sallis, and W. Brown, "Correlates of Adults' Participation in Physical Activity: Review and Update," *Medicine & Science in Sports & Exercise* 34, no. 12 (2002): 1996–2001.

25. J. L. Huberty, L. B. Ransdell, C. Sigman, J. A. Flohr, B. Schult, O. Grosshans, and L. Durrant, "Explaining Long-Term Exercise Adherence in Women Who Complete a Structured Exercise Program," *Research Quarterly for Exercise and Sport* 79, no. 3 (2008): 374–84.

Chapter 13

1. Rafaella Molteni et al., "A High-Fat, Refined Sugar Diet Reduces Hippocampal Brain-Derived Neurotrophic Factor, Neuronal Plasticity, and Learning," *Neuroscience* 112, no. 4 (2002): 803–14.

2. B. A. White, C. C. Horvath, and T. S. Conner, "Many Apples a Day Keep the Blues Away—Daily Experiences of Negative and Positive Affect and Food Consumption in Young Adults," *British Journal of Health Psychology* 18, no. 4 (November 2013): 782–98.

3. J. K. Boehm et al., "Association Between Optimism and Serum Antioxidants in the Midlife in the United States Study," *Psychosomatic Medicine* 75, no. 1 (January 2103): 2–10.

4. George Leonard, *Mastery: The Keys to Success and Long-Term Fulfillment* (New York: Plume, 1992).

5. Jon Kabat-Zinn, *Full Catastrophe Living: Using the Wisdom of Your Body and Mind to Face Stress, Pain, and Illness* (New York: Delta, 1990).

6. Sally A. Shumaker, Judith K. Ockene, and Kristin A. Riekert, *The Handbook of Health Behavior Change* (New York: Springer Publishing Company, 2004).

7. B. Hölzel et al, "Mindfulness Practice Leads to Increases in Regional Brain Gray Matter Density," *Psychiatry Research* 191, no. 1 (2011): 36–43.

8. T. Kjaer, "Increased Dopamine Tone During Meditation-Induced Change of Consciousness," *Cognitive Brain Research* 13, no. 2 (2002): 255–59.

9. M. Friese, C. Messner, and Y. Schaffner, "Mindfulness Meditation Counteracts Self-Control Depletion," *Consciousness and Cognition* 21, no. 2 (June 2012): 1016–22.

10. Ramesh Mehay, "The Conscious Competence Learning Model," 2010, www.essentialgptrainingbook.com/chapter-29.php.

11. "The Conscious Competence Ladder: Keep Going When Learning Gets Tough," Mind Tools, www.mindtools.com/pages/article/newISS_96.htm.

Onward!

1. Sally A. Shumaker, Judith K. Ockene, and Kristin A. Riekert, *The Handbook of Health Behavior Change* (New York: Springer Publishing Company, 2004).

Appendices

1.   M. Irwin and D. Hegsted, "A Conspectus of Research on Protein Requirements of Man," *Journal of Nutrition* 101, no. 3 (March 1971): 385–428.

2.   "Position of the American Dietetic Association: Vegetarian Diets," *Journal of the American Dietetic Association* 103, no. 6 (June 2003): 748–65.

3.   V. R. Young and P. L. Pellett, "Plant Proteins in Relation to Human Protein and Amino Acid Nutrition," *American Journal of Clinical Nutrition* 59, no. 5 (May 1994): 1203S–12S.

4.   The RDA for protein assumes that adults need, on average, little more than 0.5 grams of protein daily per kilogram of body weight. Because individuals vary in their ability to utilize proteins, the RDA adds 0.3 grams per kilogram as a safety factor. If you are curious as to how you stack up with the RDA protein guidelines, you can divide your weight in pounds by 2.2 to get your weight in kilograms. Then multiply your kilogram weight by 0.8 to calculate the RDA standard protein requirement for adults. For example, if you weigh 155 pounds and divide it by 2.2, you'll find you weigh 70.45 kilograms. Multiplied by 0.8, you'll come up with 56.36 grams for your daily protein requirement.

5.   T. Colin. Campbell, "The Protein Puzzle: Picking Up the Pieces," Center for Nutrition Studies, August 1, 1995, http://nutritionstudies.org/protein-puzzle-picking-pieces.

6.   Goran Bjelakovic et al., "Antioxidant Supplements for Prevention of Mortality in Healthy Participants and Patients with Various Diseases," *Cochrane Database of Systematic Reviews* 3 (March 14, 2012).

7.   Jaouad Bouayed and Torsten Bohn, "Exogenous Antioxidants—Double-Edged Swords in Cellular Redox State: Health Beneficial Effects at Physiologic Doses versus Deleterious Effects at High Doses," *Oxidative Medicine and Cellular Longevity* 3, no. 4 (July-August 2010): 228–37.

8.   H. Melhus, K. Michaelsson, A. Kindmark, et al., "Excessive Dietary Intake of Vitamin A Is Associated with Reduced Bone Mineral Density and Increased Risk for Hip Fracture," *Annals of Internal Medicine* 129, no. 10 (November 1998): 770–78.

9.   L. J. Harnack and D. Lazovich, "Vitamin A Intake and the Risk of Hip Fracture in Postmenopausal Women: The Iowa Women's Health Study," *Osteoporosis International* 15, no. 7 (July 2004): 552–59.

10. Susan Taylor Mayne, "Beta-carotene, Carotenoids, and Disease Prevention in Humans," *The FASEB Journal* 10, no. 7 (May 1996): 690–701.

11. M. J. Bolland, A. Avenell, J. A. Baron, A. Grey, G. S. MacLennan, G. D. Gamble, and I. R. Reid, "Effect of Calcium Supplements on Risk of Myocardial Infarction and Cardiovascular Events: Meta-Analysis," *BMJ* 29, no. 341 (July 2010): c3691.

12. Joseph Keon, *Whitewash: The Disturbing Truth About Cow's Milk and Your Health* (Gabriola Island, BC: New Society Publishers, 2010).

ACKNOWLEDGMENTS
AND GRATITUDE

I am deeply grateful to esteemed colleagues, physicians, dietitians, authors, chefs, and friends for their enthusiastic support of this project from its inception. Each interview I asked for was generously granted, every emailed question answered—with insights and references that informed, enriched, and enlightened this manuscript enormously: T. Colin Campbell, PhD; Dr. Hans Diehl, DHSc; Caldwell B. Esselstyn Jr., MD; Michael Greger, MD; Frank Hu, PhD; Howard Jacobson, PhD; Joel Kahn, MD; Thomas Campbell, MD; John McDougall, MD; Pam Popper, ND; Howard Lyman; Victoria Moran; Nick Cooney; Joseph Keon; Gene Baur; Stephan Herzog; Gabrielle Turner-McGrievy, PhD; Glen Merzer; and Brian Wendel.

With enormous appreciation to Neal Barnard, MD, whose far-reaching work extends to so many avenues of the plant-based movement—I am honored and privileged for all of the opportunities for making a difference that you've extended to me. Thank you to Susan Levin, RD, for your generous availability and ready answers with nutrition, and Julieanna Hever, RD, for your enthusiastic support and manuscript review.

Endless appreciation to so many in the plant-based community who generously shared their insights and expertise: Suzy Amis Cameron, Karen Campbell, LeAnn Campbell, Colleen Holland, Ellen Jaffe Jones, Linda and Dave Middlesworth, Miyoko Schinner, and Ann and Larry Wheat. Thank you also Chef AJ; Jean Antonello; Janice Bird; Paulo de Sousa; Debby Knight Fisher; J. C. Hughes; Caroline Love; Sharon, Dave, Tess, Marcie, and Evan McRae; Amy Montoya; Jim and Kathy Presentati; and Josh Tetrick.

To my recipe testers, I appreciate your patience and boundless good cheer in the kitchen more than you know: Sheri Armour, Chanda Bailey, Cheryl Duvall, Kristie Foss, Sybil Janke, Amy Shockley, Mark Sutton, and Pam Younghans. Thanks also to dear Greg for your tireless taste-testing and toleration of a kitchen in shambles. You are my best reason for getting into the kitchen.

To the hundreds of survey responders—and you may well see yourself quoted somewhere within these chapters—thank you!

To the fine team at BenBella—Glenn Yeffeth, Heather Butterfield, Sarah Dombrowsky, Alicia Kania, Adrienne Lang, Lindsay Marshall, and Monica Lowry—for your brilliant vision and collaborative enthusiasm, unique in the publishing world: thank you. Thanks to my agent, Marilyn Allen, for your passion for and confidence in this project.

To my readers and fellow sojourners on the plant-based journey, thank you. We are all on this healthy, happy adventure together.

ABOUT THE AUTHOR

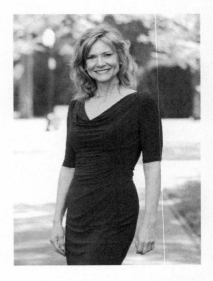

Lani Muelrath, MA, is an award-winning teacher, author, and speaker well known for her expertise in plant-based, active, mindful living. Lani has served as presenter and consultant for the Physician's Committee for Responsible Medicine and the Complete Health Improvement Project. She is published in prominent periodicals including *Prevention* magazine, *USA Today*, and *The Saturday Evening Post*, and has been featured on ABC-TV and CBS-TV, on numerous radio shows, and has created and starred in her own CBS television show, *Lani's All-Heart Aerobics*.

Recipient of the California Golden Apple Award for Excellence in Instruction, Lani is the author of *Fit Quickies: 5-Minute Targeted Body-Shaping Workouts*; guest lecturer at San Francisco State University; and associate faculty in Kinesiology at Butte College, where her book has been adopted as a required course textbook. She is certified in Plant-Based Nutrition from Cornell University and maintains multiple teaching credentials in the State of California. A Certified Behavior Change Specialist, Lani is also a credentialed Advanced Fitness Nutrition Specialist and maintains multiple other certifications.

Lani presents and lectures extensively and counsels a variety of clients throughout the world from her northern California–based private practice on successful transition to healthy plant-based living.

To learn more, visit Lani online:

www.lanimuelrath.com

f /lanimuelrath

🐦 @lanimuelrath

𝕡 /lanimuelrath

📷 /lani.muelrath

INDEX

fiber and, 48
gain, 51, 161
hunger satisfaction and, 46–47, 51
ideal, 3
loss, 3, 44–46, 53, 68, 182
management, 4, 79–80
vegetarian diet and, 21
Wendy's, 126
wheat flour, 43–44
white flour, 4, 44, 45
whole foods, 8, 27, 36, 45–46, 49, 89
Whole Foods Market, 17

whole grain breakfast template, 96–97
whole grains
consumer purchases of, 15
lowered mortality risks and, 5
meal planning and, 92, 94
Meditteranean diet and, 52
processing of, 43–44
U.S. Dietary Guidelines and, 14
workplace readiness, 121–123
World Health Organization, 6

Y

yoga, 21, 165